DEEPLY WOUNDED HOPE

DEEPLY WOUNDED HOPE

HOW GOD BRINGS LIFE
FROM
ABUSE AND HARDSHIP

by

HEATHER V SHORE

Heather V Shore's books may be purchased for educational or sales promotional use. For information please contact: Heather V Shore, 2987 Sun Creek Ridge Evergreen, CO 80439 or visit us at www.heathervshore.com

Cover design by Roy Roper of Wideyedesign
Editing by Deborah Christensen, Facets Editorial Services

Library of Congress Control Number:
TX0008191346 / 2015-09-22

FIRST EDITION
Deeply Wounded Hope – 1st ed.
ISBN: 978-0-578-19204-8

CONTENTS

To my wonderful husband Mike. You have brought such joy, fun and laughter into my life. I'm excited to spend this wonderful journey with you.

CHAPTER 1

JOURNEYS

DIVORCED, SUDDENLY SINGLE? WHAT QUESTIONS DO YOU HAVE ABOUT YOUR JOURNEY?

"If I find in myself desires which nothing in this world can satisfy, the only logical explanation is that I was made for another world."

C.S. Lewis

"**H**ERE I am again, back where I began, wandering aimlessly down a path I can't figure out. Here we go again, saying things we didn't mean, apologizing for them, and then never discussing how they hurt. This is the fourth time this year it's happened. But, my loved ones and friends don't care how it rips me to the core. How hard I've worked for the past three years to get myself back on track. Many detours along the way, distractions placed in my way, keeping me from realizing my potential. I have so much to give and offer, yet my friends don't take me seriously.

"My imagination runs wild with things yet to come, things that have come and gone, and the present sitting idly before and around me, making me want more. Will I go after my dreams finally or will I let all these people and distractions keep me from realizing them? The truth is, I can't let it or them get in my way again. But, is the way I'm headed truly the way I supposed to be going?

"This path, this journey called life that I constantly question. Everything around me makes me sit and wonder: Isn't there something more?"

That's a journal entry from 2006, after I went through three years of healing to get to a place where I still questioned the journey God put me on. The healing process from abuse, divorce and growing up can take longer than we expect, with twists and turns. Those who think healing comes within two weeks of a divorce are seriously deluded. And yet, our society seems to think we should brush ourselves off after a lifealtering change, go back to work and be OK. But what does OK mean? We all hear it—at church, home, work, at the gym, at coffee shops-how are you? I'm fine, or I'm OK. OK means satisfactory, but not especially good. Is this the life we are called to as Christians? No. We are all designed to live an abundant, lifegiving existence. We feel it in our core, otherwise we wouldn't be enamored with the underdog stories.

As I pondered the journey I was on, it became apparent I was meant to serve God, and to serve and love others with a grateful heart and attitude. That serving and giving to others within healthy boundaries was something to incorporate and live out.

As a divorced and suddenly single woman, I needed to answer several questions about the journey I was on. Was this path the right one for me? What is healthy? What is contentment? Where do these voids that I can't seem to fill come from? At what point can I feel comfortable with the choices I've made? Why does it take adversity for me to realize there is a path to all this? Do I truly forgive myself for the choices I've made? Can I rectify my choices? Out of the choices, can new dreams come and grow?

After such a big life change as divorce and sudden singleness, we are left with feelings of failure, hopelessness, and expectation. How do I align my expectations before going back into the dating world? Do I take time off from dating or jump right back in? What's the healthiest approach? Oh, and by the way, maybe I should pray about what to do. The surprising thing about the new chapter in the dating journey was seeing women who had been abused jump straight into another mar riage instead of doing the work they needed to do. Of course, I would ask God, "Why them and not me?" That was such an unhealthy attitude, but I still felt it.

The dissatisfaction in my life caused me to constantly question where God put me. It left me searching for contentment as I struggled to move into the next phase of the journey. The realization that all of us are broken, wanting and craving more than we have, kept bringing me back to one fundamental truth—God created us to crave Him. On this side of heaven, many desires will remain unsatisfied. But, God will work out all things for our good. "With God all things are possible" (Matt. 19:26, NIV). "For I can do everything through Christ, who gives me strength" (Philippians 4:13, NLT.)

As God healed me in Nashville, it became clear that it was for a reason. He needed to heal my expectations and give me new dreams to hold dear to my heart. God can give us new dreams and hopes—we just have to ask Him and let go of the old ones. And for me, most importantly as a newly single woman, I had to mourn my past in order to move forward. God replaced my past with breathless expectation of a new future. As soon as we abandon ourselves to God and do the task He gave us, He begins to fill our lives with surprises. When we have the right relationship with God, life is full of spontaneous, joyful uncertainty and expectancy. He makes all things new and His mercies are new each day. "This means that anyone who belongs to Christ has become a new person. The old life is gone; a new life has begun!" (2 Corinthians 5: 17, NLT).

As I continued on the journey, it became clear the devil kept holding me back, or least I let him. He knew what distractions would hold me back. As I met more women through volunteering at the YWCA and other domestic violence organizations, it became apparent that each one was part of a bigger universal story. We are all at war for the survival of our souls. And Satan will do anything to take us away from God. That's why we can't give up fighting or caring about others. Live each day in His presence and grace because, in the end, that's all we've got.

Remember, that we are not alone in our journey (Ephesians 3:18). The love we seek is beyond what we can imagine. Living in community is how we learn how God's love works. P. Rinehart said, "Perhaps the richest part of this journey is discovering that God is not put off by a heart in need of repair. He, indeed, sits at the foot of our bed, waiting for us to recognize His presence where we least expect it."

As each of us moves forward, what questions will we ask? What important thing is God revealing to us? How do we view ourselves and our dreams? What do we wait for with breathless expectation as we round the next bend in the journey? Each story is unique to each individual. That's how God made us—unique, loved, and special and filled with gifts. Let's cling to Psalm 139 and let that sink into our soul.

CHAPTER 2

HAPPILY EVER AFTER DOESN'T EXIST: SURVIVING DOMESTIC VIOLENCE

"It's not the circumstances that determine who you're gonna be, but how you deal with these problems and pains that come your way."

Mat Kearney

SETH

OUR first date was over seven hours long. Seth was easy to talk to, pleasant to be around and charming. We started with dinner at an Italian place, then we went hiking at one of his favorite places, took in a movie and, finally, we rented a movie. I wouldn't let him kiss me because I didn't kiss on the first date. So, he asked if he could kiss me on the cheek and I said yes. I sent him an email he next day, thanking him for the date. I had fun spending time with him. He later told me that he wasn't going to ask me out again because I didn't kiss him. The only reason he asked me out again was because I sent the email.

We met a few weeks before at a college club. I had no idea that he joined the club just to get to know me. As we talked, I realized he understood finance. His dad taught the main finance class on campus and I was failing it. I needed a tutor. So, we decided I would pay him to tutor me for a couple of hours a week so I could at least pass with C.

He came to my 21st birthday party a few weeks after our first date. I remember telling my mom, "I think I'm going to marry this man someday."

Then, he left town for his summer job at a Boy Scout camp. I went to see him while he was there and the same topic of conversation kept coming up—sex. He wanted to have sex and I wanted to wait. Every talk came back to that. He said he would wait for me, but then he brought up the fact that I had slept with my first boyfriend. He said, "You've had more sex than me because you slept with your boyfriend while you dated."

Neither of us were virgins. He pushed every boundary to get me to consummate our relationship. Finally, I gave in at the end of the summer.

Soon, our conversations turned to marriage. We would have good times together, but then we would fight about stupid stuff. I don't remember what we fought about; I just remember his anger over seemingly small issues. He had to have his way.

The need to be right were familiar echoes of my childhood. I thought this was normal for adult relationships because of what I had seen modeled at home and in other family relationships. Even the way people argued or didn't argue formed the way I viewed relationships. It never occurred to me that his sensitivity to small issues would end up being a bigger issue in the long run.

One night after a movie, he got down on one knee in the parking lot of a church. I was stunned. We had been discussing marriage for several months. He said he wanted to take an ordinary day and make it special. I said yes, but felt vaguely disappointed that he didn't seem to put any thought into the proposal. His proposal didn't include anything that reflected his knowledge about me and what would make me happy. And most importantly, he did not ask my father. My father was not happy, but didn't say anything. The pattern of not talking about our feelings or dealing with conflict was strongly embedded in my family. We just moved on without dealing with issues.

We started planning the wedding, including premarital counseling sessions at my childhood church. In one session, he described a time we went to Dillard's to register for china and other wedding presents. I have Irritable Bowel Syndrome, which at times gets irritated and I need to go to the bathroom as soon as possible. It hit me that day and I told him I needed to go to the bathroom, quickly, and I left him there. He was furious with me because he didn't know the mall, so he didn't know where he was going. Seeing the extent of his reaction to the situation, the session counselor told him to be more understanding of my health issues. I don't believe he heard a single thing the counselor said.

Over the Thanksgiving and Christmas holidays, we spent time with my extended family. After Seth's graduation in December, we went on a trip to Australia with our Symphonic Wind Ensemble. It seemed like a dream vacation. Seth was able to participate because he paid for the trip ahead of time. In Sydney, we had a horrible fight before a special outing to the Opera House to hear Die Fieldermaus. Our special picture of the outing includes me with eyes red from crying. I don't remember what we fought about but according to Seth, the incident was my fault. Everything always ended up being my fault. We enjoyed the rest of the trip because he got what he wanted. There weren't any more fights on the way back to the U.S.

Seth moved to Colorado for his first job out of college. He was alone and unhappy. We talked all the time on the phone and through email. I went for a visit over spring break. One day, we decided to go skiing. This turned out to be disastrous because it my first time ever skiing. We took lessons, but I freaked out when I got to the top of the mountain because it was so steep. He was not at all supportive of my plight. He forced me to ski by myself and I had to get the ski instructor to help me down the mountain. My fear made him unhappy.

He belittled my family. He said I was like my mother, who suffers with an anxiety disorder. He told me my parents were controlling, fearful and overprotective people. He also called my brother a mama's boy. I was happy when the ski trip was over and I went back to finish college.

During the next few months, we had fights on the phone. During these fights, he projected his insecurities onto me and told me that I was not giving him the attention he felt he deserved. Afterwards, I hid in my closet at school and cried while I tried to sort things out.

My parents didn't know him and wanted to spend more time with him, but didn't have the opportunity because we had been apart for over seven months of the 15 months we had been dating. Two weeks before the wedding, he called me a bitch. After that conversation, my mother told me I didn't have to marry him. My roommate in college did not like him. Another friend observed that his father was a jerk as a professor. But, I didn't feel like I could cancel the wedding because my parents had spent $10,000 on it.

The Big Day

When my extended family started to arrive for the June wedding, my little cousin, who was one of my flower girls, did not like my groom at all. She called him "ugly."

She was very intuitive at the tender age of 5. The wedding went off without a hitch. When we got to the reception, we did the necessary reception things. Then, he spent a majority of the evening with his family. I remember gathering at the end of the evening to go upstairs to our room, and making arrangements for someone to drop us off at the airport for our honeymoon the next day. I was hoping for romantic lovemaking on my honeymoon night and was sorely disappointed. Sex didn't last long, maybe 15 minutes.

The honeymoon turned into a nightmare. He argued with me and got mad when I wouldn't do exactly what he wanted sexually. I felt humiliation and sorrow about what I had done. It wasn't how I imagined our honeymoon. We were on a beautiful Caribbean island, at a gorgeous multi-million dollar home on a beach with our own private pool, but my husband was already letting me know how I made him mad at the slightest inconvenient thing I did.

The trip out to Colorado was uneventful. But, our fights became worse. I had a hard time finding a marketing job and was forced to take whatever job I could find. I worked at a sales job for three weeks and then switched to Walgreens to open a new location as an assistant store manager. As I continued to search for a job, I asked him where I could search. He told me the only location he would consider was Denver. He loved the west and wanted to stay in the area. I agreed to this decision.

I remember fighting and then walking around

the neighborhood of West Pueblo, staring at my new surroundings. We were going to church together but not getting anything out of it.

During college and after I graduated, I had a hard time finding a church. And now, I didn't feel a sense of belonging anywhere. I was completely lost in a place I did not want to be. My dreams of a wonderful marriage were diminishing before my eyes. The put-downs and never knowing what I was going to get when I came home were the scariest part of my new life.

My parents did not fight often, and if they did, they never did it in front of us. I didn't know what fighting was and couldn't comprehend healthy conflict resolution. I'm not sure about his parents. They argued about stuff, but from what I saw, it was stuffed and never confronted in a healthy fashion.

Colorado

I finally got a job in Denver as an advertising coordinator. The fighting continued, especially when it came to "the budget." We put a certain amount of our salaries into savings, Roth IRAs, and 401K. If our grocery budget went over the $200-$250 limit he had established, I got in trouble. I did most of the grocery shopping, but he went with me to make sure we only buy things that were on sale. He found a job in the call center at a large financial investment company. He was driven and received promotions three times in two-and-a-half-years.

The verbal abuse over budgets and other things I did wrong escalated. At first, he shoved me around the apartment into cabinets, the kitchen, the bathroom, throwing me onto the bed, and finally into the walls. Once when he threw me onto the bed, my glasses smashed into my face and I had a bruise that looked like a black eye. My coworkers became concerned. During that first year of marriage, I had medical problems, such as pleurisy, and I made a trip to the emergency room for a possible broken hand. Seth had tried to punch me in the face and I put up my hand to protect my face. It turned out that my hand wasn't broken. The first time he slapped me was in February. I just sat in the chair, stunned, unable to move with multiple thoughts running through my mind.

The violence continued with shoving, pushing me into the cabinets, and spitting in my face. I would fight back, yell back at him, call him cuss words and scream, too. This didn't make me any better than him. This was not the way I envisioned a marriage relationship. The spitting got worse and it didn't take much to tick him off. I remember him punching me in the arm so hard that I had bruises. At one point around my birthday, he shoved me into the closet, spit in my face, and then proceeded to punch me. I blocked his punch with my hand and, again, I thought he had broken it—it hurt so badly. We went to the emergency room; he apologized all the way.

I hid my bruises with my clothes-on my legs and arms. People didn't know he was hitting me repeatedly.

Then, the final straw came right before his Certified Financial Analyst exam. I knew he was going to be gone for the whole day, so I started planning my escape. Two days before his exam, he got so mad, he placed his hands around my neck and hit my head against a board while strangling me. I promised myself that was it—I had to run. He was going to kill me!

I left on June 1st, less than a year after our wedding. I left a note saying I was leaving him and not coming back. I was so upset; I stayed with coworker while I tried to figure out where to go. My coworker called my parents and told them she was afraid for my life. They knew that I was hiding the extent of the abuse.

I didn't know how to be honest and say, "He's abusing me." I didn't know how to reach out for help and therefore I didn't tell people.

My parents showed up the next day. We decided to go back to the apartment to get some of my clothing. Seth and his mom showed up at the apartment to confront us. She had flown out to counsel him. My dad told me to grab my stuff because we were leaving as Seth pleaded with us not to go.

As we were leaving, my brother came up the stairs, saw Seth and charged at him. He began hitting and beating Seth. Next, my dad joined in the fight, trying to break it up. Seth's mother accidentally got hit. My mom screamed at the top of her lungs. A neighbor heard the commotion and called the police. The police showed up 10 minutes later, broke up the fight, and had a serious talk with me and Seth. I told the police about the strangling incident. The police told me that since he strangled me, he was at level 8 out of 10 points—10 being homicide. The cop told me to go with my parents back to Tulsa and figure things out. The cops talked to Seth about his behavior, but didn't arrest him. Seth told them that he has always been this way.

On the way back to Tulsa, my mom and I got into a fight because she wanted me to tell her what had been going on the last few months. I told her no and asked her to leave me alone. I felt completely torn apart inside because our families couldn't stand each another and my marriage had fallen apart. My dad told my mom to lighten up on me and to let me process everything. We arrived in Tulsa, but I had nowhere to go because I left a great job when I escaped Denver.

My parents forced me to go to counseling and talk about my feelings, which was the last thing on earth I wanted to do. They had gone to counseling and the counselor told them that it was positive to intervene in my life to save me. I felt like my parents' actions were controlling. I couldn't believe my parents were treating me this way, especially after I had been in such a controlling relationship with Seth. I was an adult, but they didn't treat me that way. My mom snuck into my room to look at the counseling intake form to see what had been happening. How could she? She continually demonstrated a lack of boundaries and refused to see her actions as anything but justified. I felt extremely violated and we had a big argument. My dad realized that having me living at home was not going to work, so he looked for alternatives.

My cousin is a therapist at a shelter in Dallas. She and my aunt, Annette, suggested that I stay at the shelter. So, I packed up and moved to Dallas. Best move ever! The shelter was filled with interesting characters. I met a mom who was very in touch with her sexual side. She didn't care how her significant other treated her as long as she was getting sex. I also met a drug addict, and a career woman who couldn't get away from her controlling boyfriend. All wonderful ladies and I loved the group therapy sessions. I had my own room, and as part of the deal we had to clean up the shelter. Free food, a warm bed and the ability to start over.

I tried so hard to find a job in Dallas. After three months of looking, I decided to go back to Denver to finally end my marriage. I knew the only way to end the marriage was to confront him, his behaviors and our pseudo life together head on.

How silly! My family in Dallas were heartbroken at my choice. But, I thought that it was the only way he would divorce me, and finally let me be free. After driving 16 hours back to Denver in one day, I went to the apartment. He had moved out per my request and we searched for a new place to live. We didn't live together for three months as we tried to figure things out.

We moved into a new apartment and I got a puppy—my little girl. I wanted someone to love me so desperately. Nadia, my Siberian husky, was one of the best things that ever happened to me. She was a rock during trying times with such a sweet personality.

After I came back to Denver, we had a honeymoon period of three months. We hung out with friends, and joined a church and young married group. I even sang on a CD through church, which was nominated for a Dove Award. We went skiing together, bought annual passes, stayed in a lodge in Breckenridge with his friends from Philemont, and went out to dinner and movies on our date nights. I had a part-time job critiquing restaurants which was so much fun.

During this time though, I gained 53 pounds. I went from a size 6 to a size 14. I started stress-eating, my comfort, during this time. I drank and ate whatever I wanted. While fun at times, it was not good for my health. Also during this time, panic attacks randomly occurred so that I felt like I was having a heart attack.

The good news was that my husband never hit me again. Ever. But, he never let up on me verbally. It started out small at first, but his favorite thing to call me when he was angry was "stupid, fucking bitch." I began stuttering because the verbal abuse became so awful.

As the verbal abuse grew, the fights started again. He picked fights over little things. It became clear that this was never going to be the marriage union that I craved or longed to stay in. When we got into one horrible fight, I knew it was time to leave. I hit him and he got so mad that I called the police. I was worried about what he was going to do to me.

I never should have hit him because even though I called for protection, I went to jail. He didn't get arrested because he hadn't hit me—yet. I went in on Sunday and spent 48 hours in jail because court wasn't open until Monday. While in there, I found a Bible and started reading it. I also met a pregnant prostitute, drug dealers and a woman who told me how to get around the lesbians. Seth posted bond and I was out by Tuesday. I agreed to whatever my husband said when he picked me up.

From there, I got a credit card in my name, hired movers to move my stuff, and found an apartment. I also convinced him to file for divorce. I don't even remember the conversations that convinced him, but it worked. We split our possessions down the middle, but I let him have the money. Not caring, I wanted my freedom and life back. Then, we moved forward with the divorce.

He threatened to kill the movers if they took things out of the apartment. So, they brought two bodyguards with them. And, we had to have a police escort. The movers wouldn't come without one.

After moving out, I protected myself in every way, in cluding a new phone number, and an emergency plan with a woman at church. Despite this, I finally had the freedom to be myself. At my new apartment, I met my neighbors:

Rachael and her husband, Kert. She would become one of my best friends. They lived below me and we became friends instantly.

One night when Seth and I were fighting over the phone about the divorce, he showed up on my doorstep. He beat on the door, trying to get me to open it. I hid downstairs with Rachael, Kert, Nadia and Samson (the Siberian huskies). Seth finally left. Then, he found my phone number and called 21 times in two hours. I notified the police, but they said that they couldn't do anything to protect me this time. I'm surprised I didn't get a gun. I had honestly thought about cutting the brake wires on his car. He deserved to be punished for the hell he had put me through!

Leaving

During the separation, we went to counseling. The counselors identified what was wrong with my husband. I had always thought that he was bi-polar. However, the counselors diagnosed Seth with narcissistic personality disorder. Nancy, one of the counselors, gave me a book to read: "Why is it Always About You?" by Dr. Sandy Hotchkiss. It turned into my second Bible. I read it in two days. It helped me not to feel crazy anymore because it described exactly what I was going through. I started to finally feel a tiny bit sane.

Nancy helped me with so much over the course of almost a year of counseling. I spent a lot of money in therapy, but it was definitely worth it. It was the only way I could gain true clarity in an unbiased way. She helped me to get on my feet, and to gain perspective on relationships with others. She taught me how to heal, how to forgive my parents and how to let go of past situations. It took me about five years to forgive my ex-husband, let go of the bitterness and walk forward into the arms of Christ. At that juncture, I began to know what walking in freedom meant.

The more I walked in freedom, the more I heard part of me in the stories of other women. I think each woman's abuse journey is part of a bigger universal story—we are at war for the survival of our souls. Our souls are the part of each human being that makes each of us unique. When domestic violence occurs, we experience a piercing of our soul. The perpetrator tells us that our soul is not worth fighting for, not worthy of the person it embodies. It takes a person of strength, a voice deep inside, saying, "You are worth so much more." And with determination, we start a journey of escape.

Deep inside, a voice calls out, "Please don't squash me. I'm here! Please let me out. We can do it, you and me, we can make the break. The break is possible and, in fact, it's what you need to do in order to survive."

Survival, fighting for our souls, is worth the escape and making the break. The break—how does one do it and make the journey? So, here is where the story starts. As it unfolds, people can see themselves and their stories in each other's lives. Lives lived each day, with wonderful souls, waiting to be awakened, to find peace, to realize they are worth the fight.

Healing and Happiness After: Moving to Nashville

The last few months I spent in Denver with Rachael, Kert, and her family and friends were precious to me. I got to see how much fun Denver could be, but I started looking for a new job. I had always wanted to live in Nashville. I love music and was actively involved in music in Denver. I discovered that I could sing and started taking voice lessons, landing a role in "The Pirates of Penzance" and singing with the Denver Opera company. From there it seemed like a natural fit to move to a music town.

Well, God granted that wish and I got a great job as marketing specialist in Franklin, Tennessee. What I didn't know at the time was that God would use Nashville as my healing place. Nashville was where I learned how unhealthy I was, how not to treat people, how to love, how to forgive, and how to be Christ's child. I had God figured out in my head, but was dead in my heart. God taught me through relationships and my second counselor, Diane, what it meant to follow Him and He showed me how to love again. I was such a mess at times and certainly still strayed, but I tried to follow Him joyfully. The lessons learned not only from Diane, but from Nancy, Renee and many other women in Nashville were invaluable. Little by little, I dated again, learning how to love and open my heart to the possibilities He had for me.

I met so many wonderful people in Nashville, some of whom are still friends today. I lived in Nashville for five years. God used this time to heal me from other relationships I had entered into with men, and to show me how to give up control. God taught me that giving control to Him in a healthy way was better than letting a man control me. The biggest thing God did during my last year in Nashville was put me into a Bible study that focused on boundaries. An entire year—did I mention an entire year? Scott, our pastor and teacher, did a phenomenal job teaching us directly from the Bible about boundaries, and supplementing the lessons with great books from Dr. Henry Cloud and Dr. John Townsend. Boundaries are the only way to move past abuse, heal and get on with life. If I didn't have boundaries, I couldn't function as an abuse survivor.

While I waited in Nashville, God was moving everything into place for me to move to Orlando and to meet my future husband. During the time of waiting, I did question God about why others got married and I had to wait. Ultimately, God was redeeming my broken dreams and replacing them with His will. During the process, He showed me where I needed to change in order to make those dreams become a reality.

Orlando and My New Husband, Mike

In July 2008, I moved to Orlando. I had received a job as Email Marketing Manager for a large publisher in town. I fought God tooth and nail on moving there. Orlando wasn't even on my list of places I wanted to live and I desperately begged God to move to Los Angeles. I wanted to go to a bigger music and entertainment city because I had my MBA in Music Business from Belmont and wanted to work in the industry. Jesus said no and shut every door. I arrived in Orlando and started to search for a church.

Having had two wonderful churches in Nashville led me to believe firmly in church community. I saw how important that was to build not only my life, but others. I landed at First Baptist Church of Orlando (FBCO). They have such an amazing staff and Pastor Uth is passionate about living God's gifts to the fullest. People at this church welcomed me and the amazing worship blessed me. I met some of the sweetest, dearest people, who are still friends.

Life went well in Orlando and God used this time as a time to bless me with rest, happiness and dwelling in Him. One night, some new friends took me to a party at a friend's penthouse. At this party, I met the man who thought I was it—Mike. I felt instantly drawn to him and thought he was so attractive.

He said the same thing about me. That evening, we only got to talk for about five minutes. He said goodbye to me and I thought it was the end of it. I wasn't actively looking for anyone and just wanted to have fun.

The next week was Halloween and we ended up at the same party. I was a little shocked, but also surprised when he approached me. My friends said he was a baby (much younger than me) and I shouldn't consider a relationship with him.

That evening, we ended up talking in a corner for two hours. I thought it was only 30 minutes.

My friends giggled and said, "No, you talked for two hours."

He got my number during that conversation and said we should go hiking sometime. He called me three days later, on a Tuesday. I remember because it was Election Day. He found out quickly who I voted for and he was glad we had the same political affiliation because his mom didn't accept mixed marriages—Democrat and Republican. Mike asked me out and we started dating.

My prayer for Mike while we dated: "Change me and bless him!" I realized I still had work to do in my heart, especially when it came to joy. God used Mike to sharpen me. I learned a lot through this relationship and how to give it over to God. I really liked Mike and eventually fell in love with him. I hadn't been in love for more than four years, so it seemed foreign to let my heart open up.

After we dated for seven months, we hit a rocky patch. Mike decided it was best to break it off. He told me that because I was older, he always swore he would honor me by not dating me too long if we weren't going to get married. He wanted me to find someone to marry so that I would be able to have children.

We were apart for three months. During that time, God worked on my heart and I didn't chase Mike after he left. I went on my own way, realizing God had a great story to work out.

Little did I know when God said to me, "Trust me and let Mike go," that Mike would come back. He did come back, telling me he wanted to court me and eventually marry me. I was shocked. What God wanted to show me was how I needed someone to fight for me, desire me, and treat me with such respect and honor that I wouldn't settle for less. I had settled for less and it ripped apart my early 20s. Never again would I get married unless it was God ordained and brought by Him. God definitely showed up. Mike and I ended up laying all of the cards on the table and talking about everything that was important for a life together. We spent the next several months having fun together and really getting to know one another.

We got engaged in February, 2010. Mike put together the sweetest Valentines' surprise. He had also asked my dad for permission to marry him, which was a sweet gift of respect that he gave to my family and me. Mike surprised me with a camera and inside the box was my engagement ring. I don't remember much else, other than him coming up behind me and asking me to marry him. We were deliriously happy as we planned a small, destination wedding in St. Augustine, Fla. and honeymoon on the east coast.

On September 18, 2010, one of our pastors, pronounced us husband and wife. It was a beautiful, magical day that neither of us will forget. The best part was that we waited until we were married to have sex. It wasn't easy because of both of our pasts, but it was worth it in the end. This relationship was built on a healthy and God-centered foundation.

After this joyous occasion, we moved to Atlanta for me to work at WebMD. Moving to Atlanta was a mistake, especially since Mike traveled the entire first year of our marriage. We left behind our beloved church community, the warm weather, beaches and our hearts. Atlanta didn't feel like home and we had a hard time adjusting. It was nice living near part of Mike's family and we did get to do fun things with them. But, we never connected with a church, which was a big mistake. The first year of marriage was difficult because it sometimes felt like we were still single because we only saw each other on the weekends.

During this time, I was unhappy professionally and constantly questioning God's calling when it came to vocation. God gave me these wonderful jobs, which paid a lot and helped pay off all of my graduate school debt. I'm forever grateful for that. But, the jobs were not for me. As a result of hearing me complain for a year, Mike started looking for other positions which paid more and weren't in Atlanta. The choice came down to living in Atlanta or

Denver—WHAT? Move to Denver where hell on earth happened? I told God I would never live in Denver again.

Denver

In January, 2012, we moved to Denver. We both had new jobs, which kept both of us working a lot, but also afforded us financial luxuries and lots of fun. It was nice to spend time with each other and Mike wasn't traveling all the time. Then, we switched positions. I ended up traveling all the time. I would be periodically gone for several weeks, and then not travel for a month.

Again, this didn't develop our sense of team work and couple skills. We had to keep working on it. At the same time, God used this time to heal me from the past hurts and show me that it's not a place that is awful, but my choices and sometimes the people in my life that caused the hurt.

God wanted to teach me to say goodbye to the past, and say hello to my present and future. I have learned to move on from the pain and toward the love that will never let me down. Those dreams and plans I had didn't go away. They are stored inside me for a reason. Those dreams and plans, however, change as life changes. As I adapt to different situations, I can only learn to adapt what I have hidden in my heart. As I grew as a person, and gained the confidence from the journey and learning process, I realized what it took to make it and what I could do with the choices before me.

CHAPTER 3

INFERTILITY JOURNEY

SURVIVING INFERTILITY AND FINDING JOY ON THE OTHER SIDE

CHILDREN'S FOOTPRINTS

Some children come into our lives and go quickly.
Some children come into our lives and stay awhile.
All of our children come into our lives and leave
footprints – Some oh so small;
Some a little larger; Some, larger still,
But all have left their footprints on our lives; in our
hearts, And we will never, never be the same.

by Dorothy Sexton

Choices

WHEN we go through a divorce, we feel hopeless,
like a failure. We develop a "what's next" attitude.

Do I go back into the dating world? Do I take time off? How do I navigate these waters?

How did I end up back here? As we move into healing, we realize that hope for a marriage again exists on the other end of waiting. We need to mourn the past in order to move toward to our future, and our future is not bleak. Our dreams and desires change as to grow and evaluate what's important. And in doing the hard work, we are working towards something greater than we can imagine. It all contains hope.

As I moved into my second marriage, I knew what such a choice meant. It meant truly loving someone beyond me, being present, finding someone safe, and finding someone who was compatible with me, and me with him. It also meant sharing the same belief system and learning how to have fun together. God was clearly at work even when we couldn't see the ending. The love and hope we had for the future God promised us looked bright and assuring.

The first year of marriage was fun. My husband travelled for work and was on assignment in Canada. I got to visit him for a weekend when he was in Vancouver. We always had fun weekend plans because we only saw each other on the weekends. As we grew, we realized that we needed to learn what it meant to be a team instead of two independent people who happened to be married. Little did we know what hardship lay ahead of us which would facilitate growing together.

Infertility Journey

Early in our marriage, despite my age, we decided to wait at least two years before having kids. Because we spent so much time apart, we felt it was best for us to get to know one another as a couple. We wanted to make sure we built a solid foundation to base our parenting on. And it sounded like fun to wait before our lives changed forever. As we moved into the third year of marriage, we started trying to get pregnant. We had gone off birth control months earlier. I went to the doctor to figure out why an "accident" had not occurred yet because we weren't using anything. I discovered we needed to use ovulation sticks in order to figure out "when" to conceive a child. It worked!

In August, 2012, we became pregnant with our first child. I was 34. But somewhere in my gut, I knew something was wrong. So, we decided to wait until after our anniversary vacation to go to the doctor. That's when the fertility roller coaster started. At nine weeks, we learned our baby didn't have a heartbeat. In fact, the baby had passed on at least a week or two earlier. My body had no clue I had a miscarriage. What an interesting word to come to know.

It never occurred to me this could happen. And yet, it did. The wave of emotions I went through was something I was not prepared for, and neither was my husband. I didn't know how to process them. I took the day off work and had a D & C. And on top of it, I jumped right back into work because it busy and I didn't have a choice when it came to that.

No one allows a mourning time for losing a baby. In other cultures, they recognize this as a time of mourning and loss, but not in the U.S. If we didn't see the baby, why should it matter?

As I processed everything for the next month or so, I made bad food and alcohol choices. I tried to eat and drink my pain away. That's what I did with my divorce and, being an emotional eater, I wanted to do it again. So, I ate sushi and ice cream, and drank wine. It was all yummy at first, but numbing the pain gets old.

Brene Brown said, "We cannot selectively number emotions, when we numb the painful emotions; we also numb the positive emotions." It's a true and valid statement. When we numb the sorrow of losing a child, we numb the joy of living. Eventually, I felt like I was healing, but in reality, I wasn't. I had a hard time spending time with people because I found it difficult to fake it. I wasn't all right. Mike, my husband, seemed fine. He wanted to go out with others and pretend like nothing happened. I'm the complete opposite. I try to live my life with authenticity.

As we moved forward, we got pregnant again. We lost the second baby in February, 2013, and meanwhile God lined up all of these events leading into the third pregnancy which were to heal me and to move on in order to become pregnant again. My husband gave his testimony in front of church, confessing he didn't understand the depth of my pain and hadn't been a good husband to me during this time. It was a healing moment, one I couldn't forget. He admitted that he tends to tell others, "Turn that frown upside down." He didn't understand that, in order to heal, we must feel our sad feelings and that's OK.

Not all of life is happy, and if we pretend long enough, we become unauthentic. We can't take in all of the feelings at once because they will overwhelm us. In those dark moments, we might cry out because we don't understand what's happening or why. Our confidence in who God made us to be, how he formed us, and what He means to us is where the rubber meets the road. If we're honest with ourselves and Him, we go through anger, sadness, confusion, doubt, fear and, in the end, hope.

The two things He impressed on me through that entire year-and-a-half were to not lose hope and to lean into Him. When He is all we have, leaning into Him sounds like a great alternative. He waited on the sidelines, asking me to return to Him and to my confidence in what He stands for. He is the creator of the universe, omniscient, omnipresent and, more importantly, He knows my three children by name.

The hardest part of all was watching pregnant women who were due around the same time each of my babies were due. It reminded me of what I lost. At times, it was truly hard to be happy for others. But with time, I realized how much I wanted to celebrate my friends and the precious miracles entering their lives. It was a wonderful and glorious time, and I wanted to move forward as life moved forward.

Entering into a Season of Hope

As we moved onward from the third pregnancy, we entered a new season of hope. We knew we had to start enjoying the life God had given us, and to find joy in the little moments. Joy, as a fruit of the Spirit, is the one I've struggled with the most, and also the one I've understood the most. Because God gifted me with a strong will and stubbornness, I learned everything the hard way, including how to find my joy in Him.

Joy in God comes through our trials. James 1:2-4 (NIV) reads, "Consider it pure joy, my brothers, whenever you face trials of many kinds, because you know that the testing of your faith develops perseverance. Perseverance must finish its work so that you may be mature and complete, not lacking anything." Not lacking anything—meaning neither joy nor hope during this whole process. God wanted me to hold onto my Savior tightly, and to do so with both hope and joy.

We met with a fertility doctor. Dr. Minjarez at the Colorado Center for Reproductive Medicine was the next step. We explained the situation and went over my medical records. She gave us our odds, told us what tests we needed to endure and what all of it meant.

As we went through each test, we knew we had

entered a time of waiting, hoping, joyful anticipation, longing, and wonder. God kept meeting us in between: in the waiting, the stillness, and our brokenness. Rather than wishing away this time of unknowns, I wanted to be present and soak it all in. We knew we were on the right path, even when we couldn't see the outcome of a healthy baby.

In addition to the fertility tests, I had a food allergy test done to see what was causing my weight gain. We discovered I was gluten intolerant and allergic to yeast. As our tests went on, Dr. Minjarez reviewed the food test in addition to all the other tests. Nothing was wrong with either of us. The doctor told me to get off all gluten, wheat and yeast; to start taking progesterone; and to get rid of the stress in my life. This meant my job. That was going to be a huge transition.

We were left with trying to have a kid on our own or doing IVF. We told the doctor we wanted to try one more time before going down the path of IVF. In my gut, I knew that the amount of stress I was under at work was causing part of the problem. So, we waited until I started taking the progesterone and tried again in October, 2013. It worked!

Our problem was not getting pregnant; it was keeping our babies alive. We asked several people in our inner circles to pray for us because we were pregnant. We needed all the prayer we could get and we only had a 50/50 chance medically of keeping our baby. Our prayer circles prayed.

People all over the country prayed for us. Numerous times, God gave us peace during the entire process.

As a result of these prayers and all the changes we made to our lives, we had baby boy in June, 2014! And, God decided to bless us with another child, a girl, in September, 2015! Almost two years after starting the pregnancy rollercoaster, God heard our cries and answered our prayers. In his graciousness, God blessed us with happiness in the middle of the pain. He heard our cry. "Hannah was praying in her heart, and her lips were moving but her voice was not heard" (1 Samuel 1:13, NIV).

"When the world says, 'Give up,' Hope whispers, 'Try one more time.'" ~Anonymous

This quote and the hope that springs eternal in us, moves us onward. As we question the outcomes of this journey, we need to take into account what's truly important to us and what we want to happen. A good friend of mine says that God forms our families. And, she's right. God does form our families, and each family is uniquely built by His hands. No matter what that outcome is, and this is so hard to remember, He has our best interests in His heart. He works all things together for our good.

CHAPTER 4

COMING TOGETHER OVER SHARED EXPERIENCES

MEET THE OTHER WOMEN WHO HAVE SURVIVED DOMESTIC VIOLENCE AND INFERTILITY, AND COME OUT ON THE OTHER SIDE VICTORIOUSLY

GOD connected me with other women who had been abused or had been through infertility. As I met more women, I started to see patterns that centered around God's amazing love for them in their stories. Some of them had realized it; some had not yet experienced redemption in their stories and were still working through their intrinsic value in God. But, each woman was unique and gifted in her own way. Despite rocky paths filled with hard choices, these women smiled such radiant smiles

that God's healing handiwork was evident on their faces.
I began to collect amazing stories of brave women as an
encouragement for myself and others.

Dr. Mary, The Ark Retreat Center, and Laura, KY—"God Makes Straight Paths Out of Crooked Lines":

Mary went from seminary at Duke to do her doctorate
in Edinburgh, Scotland, to being a minister in Geneva,
Switzerland, where she met her Catholic priest husband.
After he resigned from the church, he withdrew. He was
angry with the Catholic Church for not bringing about
greater reformation in the church. They moved to Dallas
so he could do some work at SMU. There, Mary gained
management experience doing social work. They moved
to Nashville and then to Milwaukee where she finished
her doctorate at Marquette University.

During this time, she and her husband separated,
filed for divorce and then reconciled. Mary was offered
a teaching professorship at Boston University seminary.
He promised to find stable work, since he had trouble
keeping a job. He also tried to stop his passive-aggressive
pattern of withdrawal.

But, his anger led to emotional and verbal abuse. In
addition, he never worked and they officially divorced
during their fifth year in Boston.

From there, Mary accepted a teaching professorship

at Berea College and then became associate pastor at the United Union Church in Berea. Mary was drawn to the area and founded the Ark, a retreat center where people from all over the world have come to stay. It's a peaceful place in the hills of eastern Kentucky, tucked away in a beautiful little corner. I had come seeking answers and solace for some of the life questions that were going on at the time. I journeyed through my time there, I realized it was ordained.

My previous therapist had suggested that I get massages so I could learn what safe touch felt like. Anytime I set up retreat time for myself or needed some quirks worked out, I would make a massage appointment. The lady who massaged me, Laura, a former ob/gyn nurse, quoted Scripture about how God will take care of me: "Look at the lilies and how they grow. They don't work or make their clothing, yet Solomon in all his glory was not dressed as beautifully as they are. And if God cares so wonderfully for flowers that are here today and thrown into the fire tomorrow, he will certainly care for you. Why do you have so little faith? And don't be concerned about what to eat and what to drink. Don't worry about such things. These things dominate the thoughts of unbelievers all over the world, but your Father already knows your needs. Seek the Kingdom of God above all else, and he will give you everything you need" (Luke 12:27-31, NLT).

Laura said it took her a long time to step out in faith because she was worried about how she was going to make it. Little miracles popped up and things kept happening that showed her God was taking care of her. She asked me to give her a hug and said she wished I lived near because she would help take care of me.

These two unlikely spirits touched me during my time at the retreat center.

Nancy's Story:

I met Nancy in Nashville. We were paired together through a mentor program at our church. Little did I know this sweet, wonderful woman would be a part of my life for a long time. Nancy had two beautiful children from her marriage—Carrie and Robert. Both were highly successful, raised in DC, where Nancy worked in TV production, and were going through their own journeys. Nancy was a vibrant, lovely, Christian woman who had amazing decorating talents. She decorated her house with exquisite taste, which she shared with an adorable companion, Sassy, the cocker spaniel.

Nancy and I went out to coffee to get to know one another. After that, we studied the Bible together. I loved going to Nancy's house. We spent hours talking about how God was moving and where He was taking us. Little did I know how God would use Nancy to heal my heart from the hurt of my abuse and divorce. Nancy went through her own trial while in Nashville. As we grew together and God used Nashville as a healing/waiting place for us, I learned the truth behind Nancy's story.

Her ex-husband had severely abused her. Nancy and the children left so he could no longer harm them. She stayed with her parents for a while and eventually moved to DC for a job. For several years, Nancy was a single mother to her children. She hoped to find a Christian man who would love her the way she desired and get married again. The amazing thing about Nancy's story was her courage. She had the courage to be herself, bravely leave her husband and to be a single mom, and the courage to follow God no matter what the cost. Nancy's story is one that will always inspire me and others to live life to the fullest, no matter what happens.

Renee's Story:

Renee was my bigger-than-life voice teacher in Nashville. An established artist and regular performer with the Nashville Opera Association, she made her Alice Tulley Hall debut in New York City as a winner of the Liederkranz Competition in 1998. Renee didn't start singing until she was 29 and her talent was obviously her gift from God. The more important part of this amazing story was that her first marriage ended due to abuse. My voice lessons were more like therapy sessions as she got me ready to audition, helping me win a spot in the Nashville Symphony Chorus. The chorus was an amazing time in my life, but it was Renee who kept me grounded, sane and had my best interests at heart.

As she told me her story, little by little at each lesson,

it became obvious that God had fully healed her heart and she had guidance for me. Renee told me about how Jesus showed her the value that each of us has and how we are uniquely made in His image. Each person has different gifts and we are expected to use those to glorify His Kingdom. She wanted me to understand that God had given me these talents and wanted me to use them for His glory, not my own.

It was so apparent that despite her talent, Renee was humble. Not in the meek way, but in a way that she thought of others and her family above herself and her own needs. It taught me that I didn't have to be a doormat to be humble. When I went through abuse, I had a hard time being humble and doing what God called me to do because I was afraid of being weak and not standing up for myself. Renee taught me what it meant to be both—strong and humble in the Lord.

Her ex-husband was also an amazing singer. He played Raoul in "Phantom of the Opera" on Broadway. So, we could not sing any Phantom songs, which was a bummer since they are so beautiful. But when you've been abused, you have to draw the line somewhere. That was one of her sayings. Renee's husband gambled away their money and somehow she, too, ended up in jail. So, we had similar jail stories which bonded us even more. It's amazing how God brought these unique, strong women with similar stories into my life. It's not something I ever planned to bond with people over, but life doesn't always go according to plan. Nor did any of us sign up to wear the "abused" t-shirt.

Sadly, through my second year of voice lessons, Renee moved away to become a professor at a college on the east coast. She was such an amazing teacher. I knew she was going to bless students wherever she went. My therapist and teacher encouraged me to keep singing and, more importantly, to be myself.

Sarah's Story—A Woman I Met on the Plane to Vancouver:

I sat next to a once-beautiful woman named Sarah, who told me part of her life story: her art, her marriages, her desire to seek God, and her longing to hear the Word of God given to her by others. She explained her passion of painting and how she had a studio in her garage. She had exhibited her art in a few galleries and started winning awards after meeting an artist named Ferdinand. When she visited him, he laid his hands on her, prayed over her. After that, she started winning awards.

She had been married 38 years to a powerful man who worked for a large corporation. He was verbally abusive to her and the kids, and left several scars on their family.

But, the best part of her story had to do with painting the orphans of Liberia. She kept telling God, "Everyone is doing great things for You—I want to do great things for You." His reply was that He could use whatever talents and gifts He gave her for His Kingdom. They didn't have to be recognized by others. She dreamed of painting Liberian orphans and using the proceeds to fund a well in Africa. She went to Liberia to paint orphans. She even helped get one boy get medical care in a clinic in Indiana. Her artwork is selling and now she is able to fund the well in Africa.

Sarah also told me of times when God told her to sit for 45 minutes—to sit and be still. He wanted to speak to her. After she finished telling her story, she looked at me and said "I'm not sure why I'm supposed to tell you all of this, but that's my story." I know why—God was trying to get through to me that my service, my life doesn't have to be on TV, I don't have to be in the Hall of Fame, but I can serve Him in all I do.

Gloria's Story:

I met Gloria while teaching a Bible study at First Baptist Orlando. She was a frail and unsure woman who had suffered from cancer and numerous other diseases. She had been married to a man for 30 years who was emotionally and verbally abusive. While he never cheated on her, she thought he had and hired a private detective to follow him. It turned out that he had a Harley habit and wanted alone time with the guys. An independent man and one who didn't want to be married half of the time, he constantly berated Gloria into thinking it was all her fault. Peter had mom issues and, yet, he wanted to be a good husband at his core. His selfishness drove him to behave in unloving ways toward Gloria. It eventually caused undue stress and illness.

After Gloria had been in our Bible study for a couple of months, I could tell she wanted to change and make her life better, but she didn't know how to move on from her husband for financial reasons. Even though I only taught for one semester, the note I received from her gave me encouragement that eventually Gloria would make the best decision for herself and her marriage. Whether she stayed or went remained to be seen, but the note let me know that Christ is always at work, regardless of the situation.

Ruby's Story:

My friend, Kira, connected me with Ruby because we shared similar experiences, including multiple miscarriages. Ruby had lost one baby at eight weeks, the second one at 14 weeks, and the third somewhere between nine and 10 weeks. She and her husband went through testing to see if anything was wrong. The results were inconclusive. When I first met Ruby, they had just decided not to do in vitro and were weighing their options.

The thing that impressed me was Ruby's faith in the midst of the pain. I could tell she wanted nothing more than to be a mom again and give her daughter a sibling. Ruby kept saying, "God makes your family." It convicted me because I wanted God to answer my prayer requests my way. It never occurred to me that God had other plans, even when it came to a family.

Ruby and I have continued our friendship and it has been an honor to walk and pray for them as they find their way through adoption. It is amazing to see how God is shaping their family and exciting to see what little one joins their family this year.

Rachel's Story:

When I moved to Denver in 2012, a coworker introduced me to Rachel, another coworker who also lived in Denver. I was so excited to meet someone from my work who lived in the same city. We were the only two Denver employees for this company, which was headquartered in Atlanta. We got together at least once a month for coffee and decided to try all the different coffee shops in Denver. This ended up being a fun adventure.

During our talks, Rachel told me more of her story. Rachel and her then husband had tried for a few years to have babies. They had one miscarriage before deciding to go to Colorado Center for Reproductive Medicine (CCRM). At CCRM, she met with the same doctor I ended up seeing. Rachel desperately wanted a child. Her daughter was born through the medical support of CCRM.

It was wonderful to have someone to talk to about all of the tests, the endless doctor visits, and what doing in vitro meant if we went that direction. Rachel also understood the pain of miscarriage and could really relate to what I was going through. Rachel gave us hope because she had such difficulty getting pregnant and staying pregnant. Her courage to move forward without any guarantees the money spent would work kept us motivated to move forward. Rachel's little girl is a precious 3-year-old now; She recently came to my baby shower to celebrate our little boy.

Cindy's Story:

Another special woman I met had the opposite issue from me—she couldn't get pregnant. Cindy and I met through our church. She was pregnant at the time with her second child. Cindy and I got to know one another through a Bible study. As she shared her story, I learned that her first daughter was an in vitro baby because she couldn't get pregnant. She had four more embryos on hold in Atlanta to use at a later time. Cindy told me how jealous she felt of others who could get pregnant while she waited. She told me how hard it was to go to baby showers. She was encouraging to us because we could get pregnant so easily, but couldn't keep the babies. She was also a huge prayer warrior for us and we felt her prayers.

As we discussed how babies and pregnancy were such a gift, it became clear that God really does shape each family—whether it's in vitro, egg donors, adoption, natural or deciding not to have children. It was amazing to see how God used the fertility journey to bring us closer to Him. Because we are uniquely made, Cindy comforted me the best she could as I went through each miscarriage. She had never lost a baby, but she understood the hardship of wanting a baby and not having one. It has been and is such a gift to have friends who can walk alongside me through hard journeys.

Sharing Stories to Strengthen

In the book *The Breaking of the Outer Man and the Release of the Spirit* by Watchman Nee, the author talks about spirits touching one another after being broken by the Holy Spirit. Each story I heard from other women connected our spirits, and contributed to healing. My own brokenness is part of the process God uses for edification. "As soon as the outer man is broken, the inner man becomes strong. The wonderful thing is that when the outer man is broken, we can be strong when we want to be strong. We can be strong when we have to be strong and are determined to be strong. Try this. When we say that we will do it, it will be done. As soon as the problem of the outer man is settled, the issue of being strong is also settled. We can and will be strong whenever we want to. From that day forward, no one can stop us. We only need to say that we will do something or that we are determined to do something. A little willing and determination will bring about wonderful things. The Lord says, 'Be strong.' When we say that we will be strong in the Lord, we will become strong."

"What is a pliable person?" asks Watchman Nee. The women I've met have been made pliable. They offered up their lives for God to use for His glory. How amazing! In our culture, these women may not experience worldly success, yet their riches are far beyond what we can see. What's more amazing to me is the edification process of those who God truly loves. He doesn't leave those who seek and truly love Him alone. He wants to use us; we just have to be open, pliable and broken.

Mary lost the man she loved, and stayed to find him. Laura gave up a secure job as a nurse to be a massage therapist, not knowing where shelter or food might come from. Nancy left an abusive husband to protect her children and raise them alone. Renee was thrown in jail because of her ex-husband's behavior. Gloria dealt with cancer as a result of being in a demeaning relationship. God used each of these women's experiences to make them open, pliable, broken and ultimately redeemed.

Through our shared stories, we escaped the awful situations of abuse or learned that we aren't in control. Along the way, we learned that pain and brokenness is OK. In order to be useful to God, one must be broken in a way that can't be fixed except through the Holy Spirit. This is tough work and a realization that we don't come to on our own. Even though we aren't in control of our situation, God is in control. That is a difficult concept for most people to grasp. But, each woman shared an awareness of God's presence in the midst of her pain. Being broken is

OK, but truly learning that God's love is there, at work and in the midst of a hard situation, makes that part of the journey easier to understand and grasp.

CHAPTER 5

GRIEF AND HEALING

FINDING HEALING IN THE LOVING ARMS OF YOUR SAVIOR

"The enemy's greatest desire is to get us to doubt the goodness and the honor of God because then we will let go of expectancy and faith and hope and love."

Susie Larson, The Uncommon Woman

"No love of the natural heart is safe unless the human heart has been satisfied by God first."

Oswald Chambers

"You have turned my mourning into joyful dancing. You have taken away my clothes of mourning and clothed me with joy"

(Psalm 30:11, NLT)

THE surprising thing about this adventure God put me on is dealing with the grief in and from different situations. Before 10 years ago, I hadn't lost anyone close to me nor had I faced the death of a relationship. My life up until 22 years old was pretty good. I had no clue what lay ahead for the next 14 years. What does grief have to do with hope and healing?

Grief is a natural reaction to loss. And, we can lose anything—dreams, hopes, jobs, health, children, spouses, and even our faith. Grief is a natural, healthy process that enables us to recover from terrible emotional wounds. This is part of the healing process and there is no time table for how long it will take to heal.

Four Stages to Grief

- Shock—In the days and weeks immediately following a devastating loss, common feelings include numbness and unreality, like being trapped in a bad dream.
- Reality—As the reality of the loss takes hold, deep sorrow sets in, accompanied by weeping and other forms of emotional release. Loneliness and depression may also occur.
- Reaction—Anger, brought on by feelings of abandonment and helplessness, may be directed toward family, friends, doctors, the one who died or deserted us, or even God. Other typical feelings include listlessness, apathy, and guilt over perceived failures or unresolved personal issues.
- Recovery—Finally, there is a gradual, almost imperceptible return to normalcy. This is a time of adjustment to the new circumstances in life.

- Deep faith in Christ does not prevent grief, but it infuses grief with hope! The Holy Spirit-also called the Comforter (see John 14:26, KJV)-can give us God's peace in the midst of suffering. We will find the answers as time passes and recovery progresses. God will show us His timing and His direction as we seek Him.

Three Steps to Recovery

- Grieve—Though grief is bitter, we must let sorrow run its course. Isaiah 53:3 (NKJV) describes Jesus as "a Man of sorrows and acquainted with grief." Denying or repressing pain can lead to emotional problems.
- Believe—We need to put our faith in God's promises, trusting that our Heavenly Father knows best and that His understanding is perfect. Isaiah 55:9 (NKJV) says, "For as the heavens are higher than the earth, so are My ways higher than your ways, and My thoughts than your thoughts."
- Receive—God desires to comfort us, but we must reach out and accept it. Through prayer and meditation on His Word, we can find a place in God's presence where He will wrap His arms around us as a loving father would console a hurting child.

(http://www.cbn.com/spirituallife/
CBNTeachingSheets/Grief.aspx)

The truth is that *we* can do absolutely nothing to heal our hurts or bring ourselves joy. Only God has the power to make satisfaction a reality in our life. He is our Physician and Healer, our All in All. Without Him, nothing fully satisfies us.

Healing comes through leaning into God and finding comfort in His arms. As we come out from under grief at how life didn't turn out the way we expected, we need to pray. As we pray, we can picture God on the throne, listening to us, knowing our heart and loving us beyond our imagination. God loves and treasures us so much, and He is working out the answers, regardless of the outcome. Know that He has a plan in the works, despite the answer. "'For I know the plans I have for you,' declares the Lord, 'plans to prosper you and not to harm you, plans to give you hope and a future'" (Jeremiah 29:11, NIV). God wants to give us hope and that is part of the healing process.

David saw how big his God was and that Goliath was too big to miss. David said to Goliath, "This day the Lord will deliver you into my hands, and I'll strike you down and cut off your head" (1 Samuel 17:46, NIV). He knew he was a child of the Most High God: anointed, appointed, equipped, empowered by God. He didn't let negativity affect him. He understood who he was, and didn't complain about the situation. He walked forward, knowing he had a God-given destiny to fulfill.

As we heal and find hope, we need to trust God like David did, and not allow negativity affect us. God wants us to understand who we are, stop complaining, and change our attitude to "I am able." God will enable us to find this attitude and help us implement it as part of the healing process. We will be able to love others without it affecting us because we rely on the love of God to satisfy us. We will be able to fulfill our Godgiven destiny.

Questions to Ask Ourselves When Moving Toward Healing

1. Have I been hiding the pain of my loss?
2. Where am I in my grief? How would I respond today? How would I like to respond a year from now?
3. How have I hidden from the storm of my loss?
4. I will identify any emotional fragments, uprooted expectations or relationships in need of repair.
5. Are there others who can help me and share my load? Who are they? Anyone to help me with the journey I am on?
6. Are there specific ways I am having difficulty coping with life?
7. What steps can I take to seek help?

8. I will tell God how I feel. I will write a letter to Him and share my heart.

9. God sees beyond where I am today. He will help me press "play" and move forward. How will I let Him do that today?

CHAPTER 6

BOUNDARIES WHAT DO THEY LOOK LIKE?

WHAT are boundaries? After leaving my first marriage, I realized I had a lot to learn about healthy boundaries. What did healthy boundaries look like, how could I implement them and how on earth could I recognize bad boundaries in others? I learned about healthy boundaries in counseling and Bible study as I rebuilt my life after domestic violence. To top it off, I worked in a place where I needed to implement healthy boundaries and what I was learning.

When it comes to surviving domestic violence, boundary setting is vitally important. Boundaries are "a line that marks the limits of an area; a dividing line." Boundaries reveal who we are and what we value. When we are pushed beyond that dividing line, we end up comprising ourselves and living a life that isn't fulfilling or abundant.

There are a few reasons boundaries are important. It helps from a self-containment standpoint. They contain us within our rightful space, keep us from trespassing on others. It also helps with self-protection. It protects us from invasion and prevents others from trespassing on our physical and emotional territory. Self-protection is taking care of yourself and everything that is precious to you, and self-containment is demonstrating your regard for other people and the things that are important to them.

Once you realize that your boundaries have been violated, it is important to ask vital questions to figure out what is "my stuff"? What do I think? How do I feel? What are my values and standards? How do I look, what I do? What about my body and health? What belongings are important to me? What about my friends and family? What are my personal problems? My child-rearing practices? What are my political and religious beliefs? How am I going to develop personal self-worth? How can I develop the ability to tune into feelings and intuition? All of these questions are important to ask in order to move forward with boundary development.

Boundaries Are a Way of Life

- Boundaries are lines you draw in your life in general. Others can't cross these lines without consequences and repercussions. A boundary is not imaginary, though you may not be able to see it. It says, "This is how close you can come to me—physically, emotionally, spiritually, financially, sexually and verbally." Boundaries, if created and defended appropriately, will help prevent you from getting angry as often, because you will feel less violated, offended, abused or exhausted.

- The boundary system is a sanctuary for the soul, a place of safety and security where the spirit thrives, where self-esteem flourishes, where we learn our value and the value of others.
- When my boundaries are not intact, I can't say no.
- When my boundaries are not intact, I have trouble living up to my yeses.
- When my boundaries are solid, I can give you my best with confidence.
- When my boundaries are solid, I can practice healthy self-care and know that this will contribute to the overall health of all my relationships.

Boundaries are the life work to which we are called, as we become the unique person God created us to be. In doing so, we become the most authentic and effective witnesses to the will and work of the Lord in our lives. Through becoming our true and authentic selves, we "shine light" and "shake salt" (Matthew 5:13-14) more effectively.

Cultivating our authentic self involves six areas of development: emotional, social/relational, vocational, intellectual, spiritual and physical. Each area includes a process of learning and growing to become who we are made to be. Emotionally, we learn to experience and express our feelings in mature and productive ways. Relationally, we learn to how to play our relational roles effectively. Vocationally, we learn why we are here and how to live that out. Intellectually, we learn to think critically, make well-discerned decisions and come to our own conclusions. Physically, we become comfortable in our own skin. We enjoy this body we've been given, and treat it with respect and honor. God created each area in us, and He will help us become our authentic selves. Ask God to guide you into healthiness. He will provide a way to become the light and salt of the world.

WHAT DO UNHEALTHY BOUNDARIES LOOK LIKE?

There are several symptoms associated with the lack of boundaries or even weak boundaries. The clinical issues related to lack of boundaries are depression, anxiety disorders, eating disorders, addictions, compulsions, and other impulse disorders, unhealthy shame and guilt, panic disorders, and marital and other relationship problems. When boundaries are weak and unenforced, we feel vulnerable, unsafe, overwhelmed, anxious, and afraid. Weak boundaries can give other people too much power (authority) or assume too much power over us (control). Weak boundaries can make us think we exist to meet the needs of others while ignoring our own legitimate needs. They can also push us beyond reasonable limits and expect too much of others. The biggest symptom is being unable to say "NO" or to ask for help. Weak boundaries create chaos and conflict.

A. Unprotected

    a. Easily offended
    b. Avoidant—not dealing with people
    c. Fearful—afraid someone is going to wound us
    d. Rigid—mental situation where we begin to withdraw
    e. Ultra-cautious—reluctant and holding ourselves back
    f. Defensiveness—put up a wall, defend ourselves at all costs

B. Poorly Contained

    a. Offensive
    b. Insensitive
    c. Engulfing—overpowering people with weak boundaries
    d. Rageful
    e. Chaotic work, family—by not responding healthily to others, life becomes chaotic

f. Risk-taking behavior—pushing yourself
    on someone and being in an unnecessary
    relationship
g. Invasive—invading other people's
    boundaries. Ask the Holy Spirit, "Lord, is
    this from You? Is this Your timing?"

You will find some examples of unhealthy boundaries
below. This list isn't exhaustive, but illustrates how we let
our boundaries be pushed outside of the dividing line.

A. Telling all or talking at an intimate level on
    the first meeting; confiding details about your
    personal life to a stranger or non-intimate.
B. Hinting, whining or complaining instead of
    asking; demanding instead of asking.
C. Trying to run other people's lives; letting them
    take charge of yours.
D. Expecting partner to make you feel needed,
    important, loved or worthwhile, and vice versa.
E. Physical, sexual, emotional, intellectual or
    spiritual abuse of yourself or others.
F. Letting someone else's mood affect yours.
G. Not noticing or objecting when someone invades
    your boundaries, and not intervening when
    someone vulnerable is being violated.

Let the information above guide you as you think

through which unhealthy boundaries exist in your life. It takes time to identify, work on and move forward, shifting unhealthy boundaries to healthy boundaries. This is not an overnight process, but one that takes time, patience and work. You are created in the image of God and you deserve to retain the dignity of that unique identity. Do you want to be all God has called you to be? You decide.

Loneliness

Setting boundaries can create feelings of loneliness that can last for quite a while and even a lot of questions. Forty percent of Americans are lonely. It's important to understand that we will create reactions in others we can't control. While we walk through this process, God reminds us how much He wants to reconnect with us. There are three primary ways we deal with this:

1. We question ourselves—we think there is something wrong with us.
2. We question God—if He loves us so much, then why are we alone? We choose to either run to God or run from Him—He wants to be the focus of our affection.
3. We try to fix it ourselves. We will try to force a relationship, which never works! We can't make someone care about us. We settle with the wrong relationship. We'd rather have someone in our life instead of being in God's will—it

does nothing but make it worse. We have virtual relationships which aren't satisfying. We can also further destroy our relationships by using sexual intimacy to make the relationship work. There are no substitutes for the real thing. We try to cover it up with sedatives, which can be traced back to a broken relationship; using addictions such as alcohol, food, sex, gambling, pornography, or drugs. We can also strike out in anger toward God and others.

The cure to all of this is to reach outside of ourselves to Jesus and to other people. John 15:12 (NKJV) says, "This is My commandment, that you love one another as I have loved you." When we feel disconnected, it should drive us to Jesus. He is the only one who understands loneliness.

After going through seasons of self-doubt, loneliness or even rejection, it's important to know how to measure the success of boundary setting. Dr. Henry Cloud and Dr. John Townsend, the experts on boundaries, offer several steps that indicate if someone is headed in the right direction. To grow in boundary development, it's essential to read the book *Boundaries* by Dr. Cloud and Dr. Townsend.

Success Measures of Boundaries:

1. Resentment—the sense of frustration or anger at the subtle and not-so-subtle violations in your life.
2. Experiencing a change of tastes and becoming drawn to boundary-lovers.
3. Developing close and meaningful connections with people who have clear boundaries.
4. Treasuring your treasure—your values will start to change. You will see that taking responsibility for yourself is healthy and understand that taking responsibility for others is destructive.
5. Practicing baby "no's"
6. Rejoicing in the guilty feelings—getting around the weak conscience or overactive and unbiblical harsh internal judge.
7. Practicing grownup "no's"—helps to develop a well-defined, honest and goal-oriented character structure
8. Rejoicing in the absence of guilty feelings—with consistent work and good support, guilt diminishes
9. Loving the boundaries of others
10. Freeing our "No" and our "Yes"
11. Mature boundaries-value-driven goal setting

All of this may seem selfish, not part of your growth process, but in the world of domestic violence, it is essential to walk through boundary development. It's the only way to fight for you and your soul. It's also what God created in order to protect your unique self, the person He made you to be. Grow in how God made you; you'll be glad you took the boundary journey.

Questions for Boundary Setting Carol Cannon, MA, CCDC, The Bridge in Recovery, Bowling Green, KY

1. Is boundary setting an act of selfishness? No, it's an act of healthy self-care. As God's creation, we are responsible for guarding the gift of life and protecting ourselves physically, emotionally, intellectually, socially and spiritually.

2. It is OK for me to stand up and speak up in my own behalf? It's not only OK, it's part of being a mature adult.

3. Is it wrong to represent my rights? Not at all. Every individual has basic human rights. It is your responsibility to do everything possible to protect your own well-being.

4. It is appropriate to assert my wishes? It is 100 percent appropriate to let others know when something matters a great deal to you. To act otherwise would be dishonest.

5. Is it acceptable to ask directly for what I want/need? It's unacceptable NOT to. Grown—ups

       ask directly for what they want and need-
       children manipulate.

6. Is it legitimate to let people know how I'd like to be treated? It is an act of mutual respect. When you tell your friends and family how you want to be treated, they no longer have to guess. This works both ways, of course.

7. Did Jesus set boundaries? Jesus was a brilliant boundary setter. He established boundaries consistently, gently and powerfully.

CHAPTER 7

THE DECISIONS AND CHOICES WE MAKE

HOW TO EVALUATE OUR DECISIONS AND LINE THEM UP WITH GODLY PRINCIPLES

"Live with gratitude and appreciation. Make good choices that produce residuals."

Matthew McCaughey

"Where there is no guidance, a people falls, but in an abundance of counselors there is safety"

(Proverbs 11:14, ESV)

"We can make our plans, but the Lord determines our steps"

(Proverbs 16:9, NLT)

"I have learned in my years on earth to hold everything loosely because when I hold things tightly God has to pry my fingers away. And that hurts."

Corrie ten Boom

CORRIE'S secret was a passion for God that resulted in a relinquishment of her personal rights, which included all expectations that life should lead her along an easy path.

As adults, we need to learn how to make decisions and choices. And, guess what? We face the consequences of both our good and bad choices. Oh, my, I have made them both. When I made bad choices, my thoughts didn't line up with God's will for my life and, consequently, my decisions affected my life for years to come.

How do we learn how to evaluate those decisions from a biblical perspective? Can we line them up with godly principles in order to live out a more abundant life? Yes. Our pathway is the one we choose and God can make it right. "And we know that God causes everything to work together for the good of those who love God and are called according to his purpose for them" (Romans 8:28, NLT). God makes straight paths out of crooked lines.

Many people believe that we walk out our destiny one season at a time. And, others believe that there is no God or standard guiding them in their daily lives. Where do these beliefs come from? It comes from a heart of disobedience. We think we can figure it out on our own, and put ourselves on the throne our lives. We dethrone Jesus Christ. This rebellion comes back to us, saying, "God, I don't want You calling the shots." This dangerous decision opens the door to false teaching. We go to sources other than God. When we walk away from what God says, we think the singular counsel of ourselves is all we need. The rebellion that creeps into our hearts and minds keeps us away from God and the incredible plan He designed for each of us. All we have to do is ask God what that plan is—He has one for you.

Every day, we face decisions—decisions that affect others and ourselves. Often though, what feels like the easy decision is not the wisest decision. God's wisdom leads us to live the best life possible. He promised to give us His wisdom when we look for it. The only way to see it is by staying connected with Him. Then, we'll live the life He designed for us to live.

As we move forward, God's unseen hand moves in our life. These events are called *transitions*. Transitions are far from easy. They are also something that people run from because change is hard. But, God calls us to change because it is part of the sanctification process of becoming more like Him.

Life is always in transition. Jesus causes transformation through transition. Sometimes, we go back to what's familiar. In the midst of a transition, we cannot cause transformation. Doing it all by ourselves will not allow us to change anything. Doing it my way causes nothing to change in my life. When we end up with nothing, Jesus always gives us something. Discomfort in life leads to our growth. These transitions are uncomfortable, but at times it's the only way to bring about transformation.

We need to look for those everyday moments of life.

God will meet us in those everyday situations—He asks us to know Him in the ordinary. Most importantly, we need to change our view. Where is the shore today? Are we looking toward heaven? Are we looking at tomorrow? Jesus will show us that He is the important thing going on in the transition. Everything is possible with Jesus!

The opposite of seeking our own decisions is developing a heart of obedience and surrendering our life. The heart of obedience is worship. When we first seek our master and understand who we serve, we find true freedom. Most people are afraid of obedience because of the sacrifice they fear they will have to make. We want obedience to be better than sacrifice. I felt that if I followed God, He would never bring right spouse to me and I would wait forever. While I waited a long time, settling for something outside of God's plan left scars that God never intended for me to go through. But, they happened because of my decision. God took those scars and used them for good.

If God calls us, it doesn't matter how difficult the circumstances may be. God orchestrates every force at work for His purpose. If you agree with God's purpose, He will bring all levels of our life, the conscious level and all the deeper levels which we cannot reach ourselves, into perfect harmony. The supernatural can create something inexpressible and produce a glow we can't explain. "Then I heard the Lord asking, 'Whom should I send as a messenger to this people? Who will go for us?' I said, 'Here I am. Send me'" (Isaiah 6:8, NLT).

Victorious Living

As we learn during the transformation, God will show us how to live victoriously. The Steps to Freedom in Christ by Dr. Neil Anderson is a great resource to gain an understanding of how to live in freedom. To experience our freedom in Christ and to grow in the grace of God requires repentance, which literally means a change of mind. Repentance is not something we can do on our own. Therefore, we need to submit to God (see James 4:7). The Steps to Freedom in Christ are designed to help us do that. It is a comprehensive process that will helps us resolve our personal and spiritual conflicts in Christ.

"Victorious living is possible and available to everyone who calls on Christ. Jesus called us to the abundant life. If we don't deal with the strongholds in our lives, God may take it away from us. A stronghold is anything that exalts itself in our minds, 'pretending' to be bigger or more powerful than our God." (Beth Moore, *Praying God's Word*)

Through God's Word and prayer, we can take every thought captive, making them obedient to Christ and choosing to think Christ's thoughts instead of our own. Keep in mind, the Word of God is the common denominator in all genuine deliverance from captivity. (Beth Moore, *Praying God's Word*) "Then you will know the truth, and the truth will set you free" (John 8:32, NIV). God cares more about us knowing the Deliverer than being delivered. Remember, freedom comes through taking thoughts captive to Christ. (Beth Moore, *Praying God's Word*)

We must remember that other people have faced the same temptations we face. We're not alone. (1 Corinthians 10:11-13). We may have been victorious in a crisis, but something that appears to be harmless may catch us off-guard. "The areas of our life where we have experienced victory in the past may cause us to stumble and fall now. We must keep our memory sharp before God. Unguarded strength is actually a weakness because that is where temptations will effectively sap our strength. Biblical characters stumbled over their strong points, never their weak ones. "And through your faith, God is protecting you by his power until you receive this salvation" (1 Peter 1:5, NLT)." Oswald Chambers, His Utmost for His Highest

Victorious Living

1. We become victors through surrender to Christ.
2. We become victors by our dependence on God.
3. Victorious lives flow from victorious thoughts.
4. Thinking victorious thoughts comes from setting our focus on a victorious God.

When it comes to victorious living and thinking, Paul says, "Don't copy the behavior and customs of this world, but let God transform you into a new person by changing the way you think. Then you will learn to know God's will for you, which is good and pleasing and perfect" (Romans 12:2, NLT).

Complaining and Learning to be Thankful

There are several things that can cause us to make bad decisions, such as stubbornness and negative thinking ("Why does this always happen to me?"), but one of the biggest stumbling blocks is complaining. Grumbling, complaining, whining, etc., are all part of a victim mindset, which Satan uses to kick us when we are down. Grumblers live in a state of self-induced stress. God wants all of us to live victoriously, freely and abundantly. We can't do that through complaining. Trust me—been there, done that, have multiple t-shirts about the same thing.

I'm not saying that we can't vent to get an issue off our chest, but when we make decisions, it's good to look at all angles. Going to God first on a choice before others will always set us up to see things from His perspective. Gaining His perspective will only bring us closer to the One who created us. When we complain, we focus on things that don't go our way. Our thoughts create our lives, and our words mirror our thoughts. It is vital that we control our minds in order to resuscitate our lives. He can set us on the right path.

Brennan Manning said, "To be grateful for an unanswered prayer, to give thanks in a state of interior desolation, to trust in the love of God in the face of the marvels, cruel circumstances, obscenities and commonplaces of life is to whisper a doxology in darkness."

Giving thanks and feeling grateful despite our circumstances are part of sanctified living that only God can bring about through transformation. "Give thanks to the Lord, for he is good, his love endures forever" (Psalm 107:1, NIV). God cultivates the awareness of the gifts that arrive each day in each of us. In this process, we come to understand the marvels of God acceptance of our life story. "In everything give thanks; for this is the will of God in Christ Jesus for you" (1 Thessalonians 5:18, NKJV). Let's not be afraid to look at everything that brings us to where we are now and trust that we will soon see God's guiding hand of love in it.

Urs von Balthasar states, "We need only to know who and what we really are to break into spontaneous praise and thanksgiving." Scarred and screwed-up though we are, an appreciation of our greatness as Abba's beloved child, vibrantly alive in Christ Jesus, overcomes the sleazy sense of our seedy self and elicits the grateful exclamation, "I praise you because I am fearfully and wonderfully made" (Psalm 139:14, NIV).

Forgiveness

Forgiveness may be the biggest decision we tackle in our journey toward victory. Forgiveness toward others, ourselves and God can take time and patience. But ultimately, God wants to extend forgiveness to us. Then, He wants us to receive it and to give it to the people who have wronged us in the past (even those who abused us). This was one of the hardest steps I took in my journey toward abundant living. But, it was the best decision I ever made. All of us can make that decision today, just by moving forward and following some of the steps below.

Forgiving Others (Sowing to the Spirit)

Author Unknown

This is an adaptation of a handout I received and I wanted to share it with you.

Many believers and their relationships suffer because they have not forgiven someone. We can't control how people respond to us, so we shouldn't try. Instead, we need to focus on what we can control. Forgiveness is the foundation of the gospel—we are forgiven through Jesus. As forgiven people, we are called to forgive those who sin against us As we do, we sow to the Spirit and reap the life of Jesus. The opposite of forgiveness is sowing to the flesh—passing judgment, which reaps death (Galatians 6:7-8). At times, we knowingly pass judgment. At other times, we do it through ignorance or from a deceived heart.

Forgiveness

1. What forgiveness is not: excusing, denying, redefining sin, nor is it a feeling.

   a. Excusing: We may think we have forgiven someone when we have only tried to forget the sin against us. Excusing or forgetting is not biblical forgiveness. We may also think we have forgiven someone when we have only tried to deny or rationalize the sin against us. We'll say things like "They could not help it—they meant well. They did their best." Our flesh loves to excuse others so it can excuse itself. Other times, we may deny or suppress the reality of sin. Denial or redefining sin is a form of escape to avoid dealing with the sin against us. None of these human methods (forgetting, excusing, denying or redefining) is forgiving from the heart. People who are full of "human goodness" may choose these methods. However, these methods are not forgiveness based on the completed work of Jesus Christ. They are an attempt to forgive through selfeffort. We cannot scripturally forgive by ourselves. Instead, it must be Jesus' forgiveness through you (Mark 2:7). Many believers feel they have forgiven someone when they "feel" better about a situation. Forgiveness is not a feeling.

b. What forgiveness is: Biblical forgiveness means to release the offender from debt, and it includes four inner decisions that we don't necessarily speak to the offender:

Forgiveness is a Time-Space Choice: We need to deal with sin as God deals with sin.

Call the Event Sin: How strange that we resist calling the "wrong" others do to us the same name God calls it-sin. Could there be something in us that desires to lower God's standard for ourselves?

Stand with Jesus: Let's view sin from the position of Jesus Christ on the cross and His completed work.

Make a Choice to Forgive: "I release you from indebtedness to me. You owe me nothing. Jesus paid the price." This is a choice, not an emotion. We can imagine touching the one who offended us as we make this choice.

Then, we can allow the forgiveness of Jesus to "flow" through us to the other person.

2. How can we recall specific past events where we passed judgment rather than granted biblical forgiveness?

    a. Confess our bitterness, malice, anger, etc. that has not been confessed. Ask forgiveness of others, where needed. Be open to the Spirit in terms of any restitution.

    b. Do not attempt any self-examination. With a trusting heart, go before God and ask Him to search our past. Wait in quietness before Him. "Search me, O God, and know my heart; test me and know my anxious thoughts. Point out anything in me that offends you, and lead me along the path of everlasting life" (Psalm 139: 23-24, NLT). God may show us areas where we sinned. If this occurs, confess it to God truthfully and thank Him for His forgiveness and cleansing. If God shows us areas where someone sinned against us, we need to choose to forgive from the completed work of Christ. The Lord will give us the will, ability and forgiveness to extend to the offender. It may be helpful to imagine ourselves with the offender, standing at the foot of the cross, looking up to Jesus. As we, the offended one, touches the cross with one hand and then offender with the other hand, we allow the forgiveness of Jesus to flow from the Lord through us to the offender. "Forgive" yourself. Remember the words of the Lord Jesus when He said, "It is finished." Rest in His finished work on the cross on our behalf. Don't overlook grudges you feel toward God. We can trust God to *change our emotions*. He only asks us to obey His command to forgive. The healing and renewed emotions come from Him.

Decisions and choices—two little words with big results. They can make or break us. They can take our life to the next level or they can bring us down to a place we don't recognize. By staying on a path that God designs for us, we can make those everyday choices beautiful. Isaiah 61:3 says it best, "...he will give a crown of beauty for ashes, a joyous blessing instead of mourning, festive praise instead of despair." We just ask and He will show us.

Tips to consider when facing decisions and choices:

- Learn to wait on God. Bow in submission without any specific agenda except to mediate on Scripture, that we might be refreshed in God's presence.
- Set specific spiritual goals for the future. List

character qualities we want God to develop within us. Target specific areas of change in our personal disciplines and relationships with others.

- Make all the changes in our life we would make if we knew we had only one year to live.
- Turn from every sinful act or attitude that God brings to our mind. Let this become a part of our daily walk with God.

Prayer: Just knowing and seeing how far You brought me is freeing enough. Thank You for loving me enough to not let go and to make me one with You because I am Your disciple.

CHAPTER 8

JOY

HOW TO FIND JOY IN THE MIDST OF LIFE'S CIRCUMSTANCES

"This day is a sacred day before our Lord. Don't be dejected and sad, for the joy of the Lord is your strength"

(Nehemiah 8:10, NLT)

"Joy is the deep seeded sense that everything is going to be okay."

Pastor David Uth

"And this is a journey—enjoy the journey you are on—I made it for you."

(God speaking into my life)

"Patience is accepting God's timing. I answer your prayers in ways you never imagined.

(God speaking into my life.)

PRAYER: Please help me to develop a fresh vision for

my life, to believe You for better days ahead and know
that You will continually expand my horizons as I trust
You to do more in and through my life.

GOING through trials (domestic violence, waiting
for the right husband and infertility) ultimately
gave me a new perspective on joy. We read in the Bible that
we should be joyful, regardless of our circumstances. That
baffled me in the midst of trials. Little did I know that
God would use my circumstances to take me through an
entire season (two years) where we worked on joy and I
learned what it meant to have a spirit of joy.

Joy is a source or cause of delight; a feeling of
great happiness; something or someone who gives joy
to someone else; success in doing, finding or getting
something. Two of these definitions play into developing
a spirit of joy: a source or cause of delight and someone
who gives joy to someone else. A spirit of joy or biblical
joy is a fruit of the Spirit.

Biblical joy comes from filling the spiritual void with
good relationships, primarily an intimate relationship
with the One who is pure joy. Jesus put it this way: "I
am the vine, you are the branches. He who abides in
Me, and I in him, bears much fruit" (John 15:5, NKJV).
Most people think happiness is the ultimate feeling, but
happiness is fleeting. Happiness is an emotion, and God
never intended for us to live in that emotional state all
the time. Happiness is a glad feeling that depends on

something good *happening*. But, His greater desire is that we experience unconditional joy. Think of joy as a strong foundation that supports a variety of healthy emotions, including happiness. The long-range evidence of joy is general gratitude, contentment, optimism, a sense of freedom and other positive attitudes.

Our society, in general, is addicted to worry, as played out in our media on a daily basis. It is a common theme in people's lives, and it saps the energy out of life and emotions. Our value systems become confused and we live like Christ isn't real. Why bring up worry in the midst of joy? Because when going through trials that try our trust, we start to doubt God's hand and worry about the outcome. "That is why I tell you not to worry about everyday life—whether you have enough food and drink, or enough clothes to wear. Isn't life more than food, and your body more than clothing?" (Matthew 6:25, NLT). "For apart from me, you can do nothing" (John 15:5, NLT).

The steps below are definitely easier said than done, but as we grow in biblical joy, we learn how to incorporate these truths into our life, regardless of the circumstances.

How Do I Overcome Worry?

1. **Rejoice:** When? Always. "Rejoice always, pray continually, give thanks in all circumstances; for this is God's will for you in Christ Jesus"

(1 Thessalonians 5:16-18, NIV). How are you
rejoicing?

2. **Relax:** "Let your gentleness be evident to all"
   (Philippians 4:5, NIV). The Lord is near—He
   is in us, always here for us and won't forsake us.
   Relax—God is in control.

3. **Rest:** "Do not be anxious about anything, but
   in every situation, by prayer and petition, with
   thanksgiving, present your requests to God.
   And the peace of God, which transcends all
   understanding, will guard your hearts and your
   minds in Christ Jesus" (Philippians 4:6-7, NIV).
   How do you find rest in your life? Remember,
   control is an illusion. When we don't take the
   time to find rest in the midst of busyness, we get
   set up for future worrying. Worry doesn't allow
   us to enjoy the present, as we can see in the
   graph to the right.

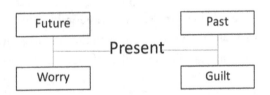

4. **Think positive thoughts—things that are
   true, honorable, noble, right, pure, lovely,
   admirable:** What do we think about the most?
   Maybes, what ifs, the worst scenarios? How

much of our energy is wasted on those thoughts? What is true about Christ and about us? If we change the way we think, we can find the peace of God in every circumstance.

Once I realized that letting go of worry was the key to knowing joy, I wanted to understand how I could get joy. What did I need to do? The joy journey surprised me because I thought it would lead to happiness and that trials were a byproduct of something I had done wrong in life. Both are misguided ways of thinking. But, I discovered one of the lasting principles—seek the only source of true joy—Jesus. Why Jesus? I often wondered the same thing as I journeyed toward understanding. Jesus said He came to earth "so that [you] may have the full measure of my joy within [you]" (John 17:13, NIV). Similarly, Jesus said, "I have told you this so that my joy may be in you and that your joy may be complete" (John 15:11, NIV). Ultimately, it's Jesus who makes our joy complete and gives us the full measure of joy. His joy is complete and whole joy.

Psalm 16:11 kept coming back to me. "You will show me the way of life, granting me the joy of your presence and the pleasures of living with you forever" (Psalm 16:11, NLT) God wants us to find our joy in His presence and in Him. He offers the fullness of joy when we sit in His presence.

We can't let our joy depend on getting all the things we want because that will never happen. There will always be something else we want. The biggest realization came when I saw that my circumstances did not have to dictate my day, my emotions or how I reacted to life. Joy does not depend on our circumstances. Again—not dependent on our circumstances. It didn't matter if I was divorced, single, married, had kids, didn't have kids, could walk or talk or see—we can live in joy regardless of where God puts us.

"True joy is a by-product of living in My Presence. Therefore you can experience it in palaces, in prisons . . . anywhere. Do not judge a day as devoid of joy just because it contains difficulties. Concentrate on staying in communication with Me. If you make problem-solving secondary to the goal of living close to Me, you can find Joy even in your most difficult days." (Sarah Young)

When we try to force doors open and make things happen in our own strength, it puts a constant strain on us and a drain on our resources. Life becomes a struggle. Nearly all joy, peace and victory dwindle from your existence. This is not a place of contentment and satisfaction.

So, How Can We Live Joyfully in Pain and Suffering?

There are several things we can do to live joyfully during the pain and suffering. We can take steps toward miraculous healing in our life and coming out on the other side.

First, we need the right attitude toward trials and pain. A trial is a painful time or circumstance that God allows in our life which He uses to change us! Trials come in all shapes and sizes—they may be small but can cause big change. The goal is to lead our mind to think of it as all joy. Joy is the supernatural delight in God. We will face trials, but joy is our choice!

Second, we need a right understanding of trials. God is making us stronger by producing steadfastness and producing staying power. Most people do the opposite; they complain, lash out at those around them, or run away from the trial (give up). God's goal for us is to grow us up. He wants to see a reflection of Himself in our face.

Third, responding with "Let" will help us go a long way in the trial. "Let" should be our response. God wants to use trials to bring out the best in us. Satan wants to use trials to bring out the worst in us. It's truly our choice in the end.

Fourth, what's available to us as we walk through trials? Wisdom and prayer. Wisdom is seeing our trials as God sees them and asking Him to help us do that. Prayer is just flat-out asking God for help, answers, anything to help us see His work in the midst of our pain. He may answer yes, no, or maybe so, but we should always ask because we don't know the answer until we ask. An example of this is in James 1:12.

Here are a few additional things we can do when we are hurting and going through trials:

- List the qualities of Christ that may be formed in me by going through this.
- Ask God "How does this pain I'm experiencing fill up the sufferings of Jesus Christ?" Philippians 3:10
- Ask God to show me His comfort in this situation so that I might minister to others.
- Living a full and overflowing life rests in the perfect understanding of God, and in the same kind of fellowship and oneness with Him that Jesus Himself enjoyed. But, the first thing that will hinder this joy is the subtle irritability caused by giving too much thought to our circumstances. (Mark 4:19)
- The extent that Jesus occupies our whole being is the extent that we will produce joy. Kindness is the twin sister of joy—we cannot have one without the other.

We can be joyful at all times, not because we are spared trials or pain, but because we are completely satisfied in Christ. Jesus promises that we will suffer. The apostle Paul assures us that being an heir of God demands sharing the sufferings of Christ (Romans 8:17). Also see Acts 9:15-16, and Philippians 3:10-11. We can be joyful, not by creating a bubbly-faced façade of happiness to hide reality, but rather by confidently knowing that in the face of suffering and trials, we are secure in Christ.

Joy is the gift of His presence. Joy is presence-driven, not circumstantially bought or delivered. We can have joy when our life is falling apart because He promised to never leave or forsake us. Joy should never come and go like money or change like the weather! He is with us every day, desiring intimacy with us. Joy knows He is with us on both the good days and the horrible ones. The joy of His presence envelops us and protect us. We need to remember that He is good and that He is with us.

"A cheerful heart is good medicine, but a broken spirit saps a person's strength" (Proverbs 17:22, NLT). Begin each day in joyful expectation and watch what God does. May joy be reflected on our face and apparent in our life.

CHAPTER 9

FREEDOM FINDING FREEDOM IN CHRIST

"The outer man must be broken before the inner man can find freedom. This is the fundamental path that a servant of the Lord must learn to take."

(Watchman Nee)

"Although it seems safe and logical to be in charge of your life, being in charge becomes a heavy, lonely responsibility. Your Father graciously offers to take your life, protect you, strengthen you, and comfort you on your journey. You need not fear relinquishment, for it leads to freedom, security and the real you."

(Cynthia Heard, *A Women's Journey to the Heart of God*)

WHAT is freedom? What is abundant living? What is making our own choices in light of these questions? Freedom, in the simplest terms, is the state of being free instead of imprisoned or enslaved. It is the right to act, speak, or think as one wants without hindrance or restraint. Living in freedom means living without the struggles that keep us imprisoned or continually making choices which hinder our life. The goal is to move forward in the different areas which keep us down.

Abundant living is the call to the fullness of life. "I have come that they may have life, and that they may have it more abundantly" (John 10:10, NKJV). "'More abundantly' means to have a superabundance of a thing. 'Abundant life' refers to life in its abounding fullness of joy and strength for mind, body, and soul." (Oral Roberts (1969), [1947]. *If You Need Healing, Do These Things*) "Abundant life" signifies a contrast to feelings of lack, emptiness, and dissatisfaction. The abundant life motivates us to seek the meaning of life and to change our life.

We should contemplate these questions as we walk through trials and tribulations. During times of hope and joy, we may ask more questions about abundant living, such as, "Am I living the abundant life?" But when trials, the shaping of our soul and transformation occur, freedom becomes important because it helps us respond to the trial before us.

What does this have to do with our journey? Everything. I realized that the choices I made inside and outside the will of God affected my overall life situation.

Ultimately, my goal was health—spiritual, emotional and physical. I wanted what Stormie Omartian defined in *Lord, I Want to Be Whole*, "My definition of emotional health is having total peace about who you are, what you're doing, and where you're going, both individually and in relationship to those around you. It's feeling totally at peace about the past, present, and future of your life. It's knowing that you're in line with God's ultimate purpose for you and being fulfilled in that. When you have that kind of peace and you no longer live in emotional agony, then you are a success." This meant learning about abundant living in Christ and how to walk forward in freedom. Only through Jesus Christ could I find true freedom.

What Does It Mean to Find Freedom in Christ?

Jesus Christ brings true freedom and He came to set us free. That was the reason for His death on the cross. He was the atoning sacrifice for our sins so that we may join the Father in heaven. The writer of Hebrews tells us that Jesus "shared in their humanity so that by his death he might break the power of him who holds the power of death—that is, the devil—and free those who all their lives were held in slavery by their fear of death" (Hebrews 2:14-15, NIV). Christians are called to liberty in Christ, receiving forgiveness of their sins through Christ's shed blood, the indwelling of the Holy Spirit, an awareness of the truth of God, and, as a free gift, the hope of eternal life.

We have a new identity in Christ when we become a Christian. Learning this new identity and applying God's truths can guide our direction and help move us to do the right thing when we face trials. Our identity means that we are children of God and we are in Christ. In our deepest identity, we are also a saint, a child born of God, a divine masterpiece, a child of light, a citizen of heaven. (Beth Moore, *Praying Gods Word*) "Therefore, if anyone is in Christ, he is a new creation; old things have passed away; behold, all things have become new" (2 Corinthians 5:17, NKJV).

We can relish the fact that we are a new creation and the old is gone. How do we apply this to our lives? Through God's truth and the Holy Spirit.

Freedom in God's Truth

Look to God's truth in Scripture to find freedom. His words offer sovereign truths which can break us free from the bondage of this world. "It is for freedom that Christ has set us *free*. Stand firm, then, and do not let yourselves be burdened again by a yoke of slavery" (Gal. 5:1, NIV, emphasis added). As we study His Word and look for freedom, we will discover a few truths to help us along our journey: Christ came to set us free, He binds up the brokenhearted and He reveals Himself to those who choose to follow Him.

Christ came to set us free. Let's unpack that. We have been set free from sin by the Son of God, who said, "If the Son sets you free, you will be free indeed" (John 8:36, NIV). Now, we can truly say, along with Paul, "... through Christ Jesus the law of the Spirit who gives life has set you free from the law of sin and death" (Romans 8:2, NIV). We now know the truth and that truth has set us free (Romans 8:32). As we can see in those verses, God's goal in sending His son was true repentance and freedom. By accepting Christ as our Savior, we can find freedom. God calls us to walk in the newness of life.

Christ binds up the brokenhearted. One of my favorite verses says, "He heals the brokenhearted and binds up their wounds" (Psalm 147:3, NIV). God's love is the salve on our wounds. He wants to wrap us up in His arms and love us through our good times and bad. He knew this life would be hard. He said, "These things I have spoken to you, that in Me you may have peace. In the world you will have tribulation; but be of good cheer, I have overcome the world" (John 16:33, NKJV). Scripture promises that trials will be a part of the Christian walk. Yet when someone goes through a tragedy or hard time, we often find it difficult to walk alongside them or give them comforting words. Why?

Most people have great intentions, but say the wrong thing. Or, they quote sayings or Scripture at us, thinking it will help us in our situation. *Binding up* means to carefully and gently wrap up or bandage. To bind properly, it takes time. To heal takes time. "Isaiah 61:1 (NASB) paints a powerful portrait of God's heart: "The Spirit of the Lord

God is upon me, because the Lord has anointed me to bring good news to the afflicted; He has sent me to bind up the brokenhearted . . ."

"Jesus was anointed to bind up the brokenhearted—but we often find it hard to love each other when we see weakness or sin." (Melody Green, Last Day Ministries) God is our healer and the redeemer of our souls. Let us be tender with the bruised and downtrodden. We don't know their story until they tell us. He will bind them properly; it may take longer than we think.

One of God's goals is to open our eyes to the truth. He reveals Himself to those who choose to follow Him. God's precepts or truths are there for us to consume and understand. "I will walk about in freedom, for I have sought out your precepts" (Psalm 119:45). As we move forward in freedom, studying God's Word is essential to finding Him and ourselves. Doing Bible studies such as *Breaking Free* by Beth Moore or reading her book, *Praying God's Word*, will educate us in the truth that is available. God wants to reveal Himself to us. Let him by meditating on what He says about our freedom.

Freedom Through the Holy Spirit

The Trinity is comprised of three Persons—the Father, the Son and the Holy Spirit. The Holy Spirit is our Comforter who indwells us. God sends Him as a gift when we accept Christ. Most people think of Him as our conscience. The Holy Spirit guides us into wholeness and oneness with Christ. He is the one who accomplishes transformation in us. God's Spirit guides us to truth (John 16:13) and helps us understand the Scriptures (1 Corinthians 2:10-14). The spiritual understanding we gain from Him can help lead to freedom.

The Holy Spirit accomplishes wholeness in us. When we tell God that we want His ways to become our ways, we can move into all the wholeness He has for us. Let's pray, "Lord, I want to be whole."

Why go into this discussion on freedom? Freedom in Christ is fundamental to growing, living with hope and advancing in life. It's important to recognize, act and grow in this area. Freedom in Christ truly does unlock the key to an abundant life, and it's something that Christ calls us to as His followers.

The goals of breaking free are below and something to consider incorporating into our daily life.

Goals of Breaking Free:

1. Recognize the sin—recognize what it is, ask God to help us discover the current strongholds in our life.
2. Pray over our weakness toward sin.
3. Claim victory.
4. Change our behavior, thoughts and speech.
5. Seek the Lord in Scripture daily. We need spiritual feeding every day.
6. Seek out a mentor.

7. Surround ourselves with like-minded friends.

How to Maintain Our Freedom

Two books deal with maintaining our freedom once we become a new creation in Christ: *Walking in Freedom,* a 21-day devotional and *Living Free in Christ.* Both are by Neil Anderson. Maintaining our freedom is important as we grow. The steps below can help us keep daily freedom a reality:

1. Get involved in a loving, caring church fellowship where we can be open and honest with others, and where God's truth is taught with grace.

2. Read and meditate on the Bible daily. Memorize key verses from the *Steps to Freedom in Christ* by Neil Anderson. You may want to read the "Statement of Truth" out loud daily and study the verses mentioned.

3. Learn to take every thought captive to the obedience of Christ. We can assume responsibility for our thought life. We need to make sure our mind doesn't become passive. That means, reject all lies, choose to focus on the truth, and stand firm in our true identity as a child of God in Christ.

4. Don't drift back to old patterns of thinking, feeling and acting. This can easily happen if

we become spiritually and mentally lazy. If we are struggling with walking in the truth, we can openly share our battles with a trusted friend who will pray for us and encourage us to stand firm.

5. We can't expect other people to fight our battles for us, however. They can help us, but they can't think, pray, read the Bible or choose the truth for us.

6. Commit ourselves to daily prayer. Prayer demonstrates a life of trusting in and depending on God. We can sincerely pray the prayers you'll find in the appendix often and with confidence. Feel free to change them to make them your prayers.

The Bible offers a unique perspective. It shows us that true freedom is found by obeying God, and not living according to our desires. The psalmist celebrated God's Word as the key to personal liberty. Psalm 119:32 says, "I run in the path of your commands, for you have broadened my understanding." Imagine what it would be like to be released from our biggest worries and to run free. It can happen. True freedom is not found by choosing our own way, but by yielding to God's way.

CHAPTER 10

HOPE

LEARNING HOW TO HOPE AND LEAN INTO CHRIST

"All it takes is one bloom of hope to make a spiritual garden."

Tern Guillemets

"Pray for a revitalization of God's vision for your life, enterprise and family."

Joel Osteen

WHAT HOPE IS

AS I continue on my journey, my focus is on hope. Hope is defined as a feeling of expectation and desire for a certain thing to happen or a feeling of trust. In the Bible, hope carries a similar meaning. It centers around the anticipation of a favorable outcome under God's guidance (Holman Bible Dictionary). My favorite definition is "to await." Wait for what?

God made it clear that our waiting time would not

be wasted. Psalm 5:3 (NIV) says, ". . . in the morning I lay my requests before you and wait expectantly." Waiting is holding on; praying expectantly; and listening to the still, small voice in our heart. Through all our choices and hardships, hope exists and will be there at the end of the journey. God wants to redeem every bad choice and decision with the hope of our future.

Stories Don't Always Work Out, But Hope Never Fails

"Sometimes in tragedy we find out life's purpose—the eye sheds a tear to find its focus."

(Robert Brault)

So many people don't make it to the other side of brokenness, waiting and stillness with the desired answer to prayer. They end up with a different story—a story they didn't plan for. It's either a story they don't want as their own or it's one of disbelief. To those stories, we should respond with empathy. Our society lacks empathy and compassion, but we desperately need them for others and ourselves when life doesn't turn out the way we expected. We can't understand why everyone's story or choices don't end up with the happy ending.

I have met many women who won't leave their abusive situation. What about the friend who has been trying to get pregnant for several years but it still hasn't happened? Think of all the other people who face pain. And yet, that doesn't mean we give up hope. Regardless of the outcome, God is there. He tells us to stop all of our striving and watch to see what He will do. "I consider that our present sufferings are not worth comparing with the glory that will be revealed in us." (Romans 8:18, NIV).

Courage underlies these stories. It takes courage to put one foot in front of the other. It takes courage to pack up and leave the one you claimed to love but who shows you he doesn't love you back through his actions. It takes courage to continue trying to get pregnant, never knowing if "this time" will be it. It takes courage to love your neighbor as yourself. And it takes courage to live out your faith, with each passing day.

Winston Churchill said, "Courage is going from failure to failure without ever losing enthusiasm." Not losing enthusiasm and hope in the midst of the story is where we develop true courage. Courage keeps us moving forward toward hope. Am I courageous enough to act like a complete person? Courage is taking a risk toward a new opportunity. Through faith, courage and hope, we can create a new story out of our life.

Courage and hope remind us that our circumstances don't need to change; it's us who need to change. Sometimes, to change us, God allows us to go through the worst things possible. After losing our third baby, I wrote in my journal, "One thing is clear, You don't want me to lose hope. You knit these little ones together in my womb and they were too beautiful to grace this earth. Somewhere in the midst of this journey, You will use this pain to help someone else. We are to lean into You and not lose hope!"

Sometimes, we want the easier journey. We look at other people's lives and they appear easier than ours. Then, God calls us to walk alongside Him on our journey so we can see His sovereignty. Whether it's a test, a trust-building exercise or a trial that draws us closer to Him through it, look to the cross. God brings beauty out of the pain and allows us to keep moving toward a better future. Lean into the Lord when hope wanes. Maybe redemption is waiting in the wings.

Faith looks back and draws courage; hope looks ahead and keeps desire alive. In the meantime, we need one more thing for our journey. We have to step back and ask, "What is all this for?" The resurrection of our heart, the discovery of our role in the larger story, entering into the sacred romance with our Savior—why do we pursue these things? If we seek all of this for our own sake, we're right back where we started: lost in our own story. Jesus said that when a person lives merely to preserve his life, he eventually loses it altogether. Rather, He said, we need to give our life away and discover life as it was always meant to be.

"Self-help is no help at all. Self-sacrifice is the way, my way, to finding yourself, your true self" (Matt. 16:25, The Message). "Self-preservation, the theme of every small story, violates the Trinity, whose members live to bring glory to each other. The road we travel will take us into the battle to restore beauty in all things, chief among them the hearts of those we know. We grow in glory so that we might assist others in doing so; we give our glory to increase theirs. In order to fulfill the purpose of our journey, we will need a passion to increase glory; we will need love. Memory, imagination, and a passion for glory—we must keep these close at hand if we want to see the journey to its end. But, the road is not entirely rough. We will find oases along the way. It would be a dreadful mistake to assume that our Beloved is waiting for us only at the end of the road. Our communion with Him sustains us along our path."

Above is writing from Jon Eldridge. Jon illustrates the hope for tomorrow because it reveals our journey's purpose. In order to live out our hope and not let go, we have to take hold of memory, imagination, and a passion for glory. Only then can we move forward into the freedom Christ calls us to. Abundant living is ours, it's for the taking. We just have to reach out and grab it.

God brought me full circle, and now, I'm ready to step forward to the next bend in the road. I am excited at how God answered prayer, made me wait and provided answers. And funny to me, how He works all things for good—including the path I've chosen. It all winds back to Him.

APPENDIX

I N counseling and other types of therapies, counselors help you identify the issues in your life. Given the emphasis on decisions and choices, I thought it would be good to include some resources that one of my counselors gave me. I am not a certified counselor, so I am passing on their wisdom. You may or may not deal with distorted thinking and how those perceptions can cloud your reality, but understanding how you think can help you unlock your future and lead you to a path of freedom.

Distorted thinking:

How you perceive *external events* (things you can't control) cause you to evaluate those *internal events* (you can control this) in four steps.

1. Thoughts—positive or negative, understand the filter with which you process your thoughts
2. Emotions—learn to not act on emotions
3. Behaviors—actions
4. Consequences

When you process your thoughts, you look at the

situation, your emotions get triggered, your thoughts follow and you make a rational response.

There are a few ways you can distort your thinking when evaluating and processing from the external event to the internal event.

1. All-or-Nothing Thinking: This is black-and-white thinking. It does not allow any gray into the decision.
2. Overgeneralization: Comes with a negative thought, such as defeating yourself.
3. Discounting the Positive: It's not giving yourself credit for things you do well, not seeing yourself for what you are. For example, tell yourself out loud that you are beautiful while looking into the mirror.
4. Jumping to Conclusions:
   a. Mind Reading: This is imagining something that may or may not happen.
   b. Reflective and Active Listening

5. Shoulds, Woulds, Coulds: These verbs and adjectives make you pastand future-focused, instead of present-focused.
   You need to eliminate them from your vocabulary.
6. Labeling

7. Blame Game: It is blaming yourself or others, and can be caused by a lack of self-esteem.

8. Self-Esteem Cup: God is the only one who can fill it up. Don't rely on others to fill your cup.

What role are you playing in the conversations that you have this week? What do you learn from your mistakes? Your mind doesn't have the concept of time and you will need to recognize if your mind isn't letting go. Positive thinking is viewing mistakes as opportunities to learn.

Self-Defeated Model

This occurs when people knowingly do things that cause them to fail or bring them trouble.

- To overcome self-defeating behaviors, do a self-concept inventory.

  - Who am I?
  - What do I like about myself?
  - What traits do I possess that make me attractive to others—how do other people see me?
  - Get to know yourself before getting to know others.
  - Look at your character traits. What you are, what you can do? This is it, this is me.

- What would you like to improve about yourself as a person? You are the only one. This is it. You need to work on yourself.
- What is my mission in life? What are my beliefs—what do I stand for?
- An example of something self-defeating is negative selftalk. This came from perfection for me.
- You can fly as high as you want—the negative thinking cuts you down.
- You can change your attitude. If your mood is affected by others, you are giving them control.

Reflective Listening

This allows you to process what others are saying without letting it influence your internal events. Reflective listening is important for relationships—either personal or professional. A few things to key in on are the different cues, listed below, which people give you:

1. Verbal: words you say
2. Non-Verbal: a person's body language
3. Paraverbal: a person's pitch, tonality, volume
4. Taking your emotions out of it when listening to others

To reiterate, here are key phrases to use when you are not sure you understand what someone is saying to you:

1. So, what you are saying is…
2. I'm hearing you saying…
3. It sounds like…
4. If I understand you correctly, what you're saying…

Statement of Truth (Bondage Breaker by Neil Anderson)

1. I recognize that there is only one true and living God who exists as the Father, Son and Holy Spirit. He is worthy of all honor, praise and glory as the One who made all things and holds all things together. (Exodus 20:2-3; Colossians 1:16-17)

2. I recognize that Jesus Christ is the Messiah, the Word who became flesh and dwelt among us. I believe that He came to destroy the works of the devil, and that He disarmed the rulers and authorities and made a public display of them, having triumphed over them. (John 1:1, 14; Colossians 2:15; 1 John 3:8)

3. I believe that God demonstrated His love for me in that while I was still a sinner, Christ died for me. I believe that He delivered me from the domain of darkness and transferred me to His kingdom, and in Him I have redemption, the

forgiveness of sins. (Romans 5:8; Colossians 1:13-14)

4. I believe that I am now a child of God and that I am seated with Christ in the heavenlies. I believe that I was saved by the grace of God through faith, and that it was a gift and not a result of any works on my part. (Ephesians 2:6, 8-9; 1 John 3:1-3)

5. I choose to be strong in the Lord and in the strength of His might. I put no confidence in the flesh, for the weapons of warfare are not of the flesh, but are divinely powerful for the destruction of strongholds. I put on the full armor of God. I resolve to stand firm in my faith and resist the evil one. (2 Corinthians 10:4; Ephesians 6:10-20; Philippians 3:3)

6. I believe that apart from Christ I can do nothing, so I declare my complete dependence on Him. I choose to abide in Christ in order to bear much fruit and glorify my Father. I announce to Satan that Jesus is my Lord. I reject any and all counterfeit gifts or works of Satan in my life. (John 15:5, 8; 1 Corinthians 12:3)

7. I believe that the truth will set me free and that Jesus is the truth. If He sets me free, I will be free indeed. I recognize that walking in the light is the only path of true fellowship with God and me. Therefore, I stand against all of Satan's

deception in taking every thought captive in obedience to Christ. I declare that the Bible is the only authoritative standard for truth and life. (John 8:32, 36; 14:6; 2 Corinthians 10:5; 2 Timothy 3:15-17; 1 John 1:3-7)

8. I choose to present my body to God as a living and holy sacrifice and the members of my body as instruments of righteousness. I choose to renew my mind by the living Word of God in order that I many prove that the will of God is good, acceptable and perfect. I put off the old self with its evil practices and put on the new self. I declare myself to be a new creation in Christ. (Romans 6:13; 12:1-2; 2 Corinthians 5:17; Colossians 3:9-10)

9. By faith, I choose to be filled with the Spirit so that He can guide me into all truth. I choose to walk by the Spirit so that I will not gratify the desires of the flesh. (John 16:13; Galatians 5:16; Ephesians 5:18)

10. I renounce all selfish goals and choose the ultimate goal of love. I choose to obey the two greatest commandments: love the Lord my God with all my heart, soul, mind and strength; and love my neighbor as myself. (Matthew 22:37-39; 1 Timothy 1:5)

11. I believe that the Lord Jesus has all authority in heaven and on earth, and He is the head over

every power and authority. I am complete in Him. I believe that Satan and his demons are subject to me in Christ since I am a member of Christ's body. Therefore, I obey the command to submit to God and resist the devil, and I command Satan in the name of Jesus Christ to leave my presence. (Matthew 28:18; Ephesians 1:19-23; Colossians 2:10; James 4:7)

"In Christ" Identity Scriptures

I renounce the lie that I am rejected, unloved, dirty or shameful because in Christ, I am completely accepted. God says:

- I am God's child (John 1:12)
- I am Christ's friend (John 15:5)
- I have been justified through faith (Romans 5:1)
- I am united with the Lord and I one with Him in spirit (1 Corinthians 6:17)
- I have been bought with a price: I belong to God (1 Corinthians 6:19-20)
- I am a member of Christ's body (1 Corinthians 12:27)
- I am a saint, a holy one (Ephesians 1:1)
- I have been adopted as God's child (Ephesians 1:5)
- I have direct access to God through the Holy Spirit (Ephesians 2:18)

- I have been redeemed and forgiven of all my sins (Colossians 1:14)
- I am complete in Christ (Colossians 2:10)

I renounce the lie that I am guilty, unprotected, alone, or abandoned because in Christ, I am totally secure. God says:

- I am free from condemnation forever (Romans 8:1-2)
- I am assured that all things work together for good (Romans 8:28)
- I am free from any condemning charges against me (Romans 8:31V34)
- I cannot be separated from the love of God (Romans 8:35-39)
- I have been established, anointed, and sealed by God (2 Corinthians 1:21-22)
- I am confident that the good work God began in me will be perfected in the end (Philippians 1:6)
- I am a citizen of heaven (Philippians 3:20)
- I have not been given a spirit of fear, but of power, love and self-discipline (2 Timothy 1:7)
- I can find grace and mercy in a time of need (Hebrews 4:16)
- I am born of God and the evil one cannot touch me (1 John 5:18)

I renounce the lie that I am worthless, inadequate, helpless or hopeless because in Christ, I am deeply significant. God says:

- I am the salt of the earth and the light of the world (Matthew 5:13-14)
- I am a branch of the true vine, Jesus, a channel of His life (John 15: 1, 5)
- I have been chosen and appointed by God to bear fruit (John 15:16)
- I am a personal, Spirit-empowered witness of Christ to share the Good News with others (Acts 1:8)
- I am a temple of God (1 Corinthians 3:16)
- I am a minister of reconciliation for God (2 Corinthians 5:17-21)
- I am God's coworker (2 Corinthians 6:1)
- I am seated with Christ in the heavenly realm (Ephesians 2:6)
- I am God's workmanship, created for good works (Ephesians 2:10)
- I may approach God with freedom and confidence (Ephesians 3:12)
- I can do all things through Christ who strengthens me (Philippians 4:13)
- I am not the great "I am," but by the grace of God I am what I am (Exodus 3:14; John 8:24, 28, 58; 1 Corinthians 15:10):2